TEETH FOR YOUR LIFETIME

A complete, easy-to-read, and understandable guide to a lifetime of dental health

by

Irwin B. Golden, DDS, FAGD

Counterpoint Publications, Upland, California

Printed in the United States of America

ISBN 0-9636047-0-8
Library of Congress Catalog Card Number 93-070966

Published by:
Counterpoint Publications
155 East "C" Street, Suite D
Upland, California 91786 U.S.A.

DEDICATED
to the memory of
Charles E. Stuart, DDS
teacher, scientist
and humanitarian

CONTENTS

ILLUSTRATIONS

ABOUT THE AUTHOR

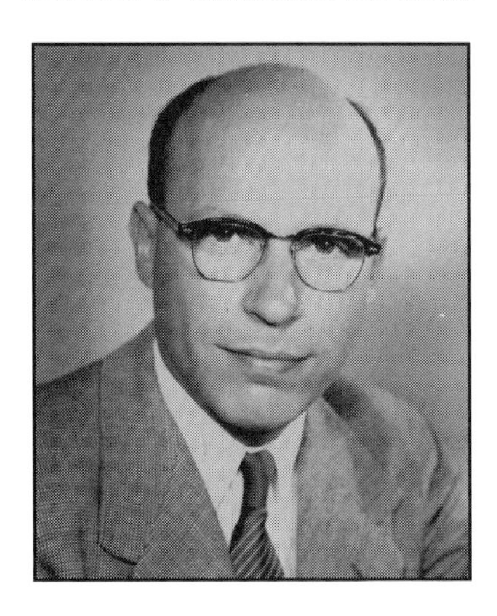

IRWIN B. GOLDEN, DDS, FAGD

Dr. Golden writes from fifty years of experience in private practice. An honors graduate of the University of Pennsylvania School of Dental Medicine in 1936, he left his fledgling dental practice in 1941 to serve five years as a Captain in the U.S. Army Dental Corps. His current dental practice is located in the Ontario/Upland area of Southern California, where he started in 1947. He has taught undergraduate students part-time at Loma Linda University School of Dentistry as Assistant Professor of Restorative Dentistry. At the University of Southern California School of Dentistry he started the Orthognathic Seminar, which he served as Director for ten years in the Continuing Education Department. Dr. Golden has five research papers published in the dental literature, has co-authored with Dr. Charles E. Stuart "The History of Gnathology," and founded two newsletters for dental organizations, which he edited for ten years.

The first wealth is health.

—Ralph Waldo Emerson
"The Conduct of Life"

PREFACE

During his excellent clinical experience for more than half a century, the author placed high emphasis on helping his patients and other friends learn more about the benefits of good dental health. His most penetrating hope was that *his* patients would learn and fully believe that teeth and their support structures represent a lifetime treasure . . . not something to be given up easily. The notion that dental problems should be solved by extraction and replacement of teeth is anathema to all good dentists; the fallacy of such treatment should become just as obvious to patients.

But dentists and their office staff members may find that some patients are not easily receptive to this idealistic message—the natural wariness of a new dental office client to what he or she may perceive as "sales talk" may be an obstacle to learning the truth about dental health maintenance and preventive dentistry for such persons. This book is "easy reading," and helps to put the message of dental health in non-promotional terms that can be easily understood by all readers.

Dr. Golden's book, from title to last page, is

directed toward this goal: helping patients and their friends and families understand the importance and practical feasibility of keeping their teeth, and maintaining the health and function of the oral environment. What a convenient teaching aid he offers to dental patients, to young people who may be contemplating careers as dentists or dental hygienists, and to the families of patients currently experiencing or anticipating dental treatment procedures. It is an appropriate symbolic climax to highlight the career of a dentist whose lifetime has been characterized by the pursuit of excellence in learning and in dental practice.

—Judson Klooster, DDS, Dean
Loma Linda University School of Dentistry

ACKNOWLEDGEMENTS

Fifty years of dental practice is a learning experience that must be credited to my patients. Their loyalty and acceptance of my suggestions have taught me that with mutual cooperation and sincere efforts most people can retain their natural teeth for their lifetime. Many of these patients have proven that it is possible to overcome serious dental problems and still achieve that goal. To them I owe a special debt of gratitude; they are living proof that no matter how hopeless the problems may seem, modern dental procedures are available to deal with them.

Among all my teachers a few stand out as influences in my career. Most notable is my father, Morris H. Golden, DDS, whose love and dedication to his profession motivated me to become a dentist. John Metcalf, DDS, whose model was Michelangelo, taught me that "Trifles make perfection, but, perfection is no trifle." Dr. Michael Walsh taught the importance of nutrition to health, and that "You are what you eat" in the 1950's, long before its current popularity. Milus House, DDS, taught the importance of retaining natural teeth because he had to learn all about dentures from personal experience as a result of dental ignorance in his day. Charles Stuart, DDS, taught dentists worldwide the principles of dental occlusion and the importance of normal function to the longevity of the dentition. He integrated the knowledge about the interaction of the temporomandibular joints and the teeth and with the help of Drs. Beverly McCollum and Harvey Stallard created the subject of gnathology as an integral part of dental science. To Andrew J. Galambos, who is not a dentist, I must express my gratitude for a deeper understanding of human values, right and wrong, and the importance of the long-term view.

For their help in editing and their critical evaluation I am deeply indebted to Max Crigger, DDS, Professor, Department of Graduate Periodontology, Loma Linda University School of Dentistry; to my son, Gregory S. Golden, DDS; to my dental assistant of twenty years, Mrs. Shelby Smarte, and to her husband, Gene, whose professional editing skills were invaluable. Thanks also to Nancy Rice for her contributions to design and layout. The suggestions of Russell R. Langenbeck, DDS, and John Conard Brown, DDS, FAGD, who read the manuscript, also are greatly appreciated. My wife Mary Anne, my dental assistant for the first 35 years of my practice, has been, and still is, the loving inspiration for my continuing efforts to educate our patients and guide them to a lifetime of health. ✤

INTRODUCTION

Is your smile important to your self-esteem? Does recurrent pain or sensitivity detract from the enjoyment of your food? The answers to these questions will determine the care you give to your teeth. And the answers you give to the Dental Longevity Test will help predict how long you will keep your natural teeth.

The notion that old age and dentures (false teeth) go together is out of date. Most people keep some of their natural teeth for their lifetime. But with average life spans increasing and more people living into their nineties, retaining natural teeth becomes a challenge. Your early and persistent efforts to achieve this goal will seriously affect the quality of your life in later years. The old adage, "Brush your teeth twice a day; see your dentist twice a year" is just not enough. Adopting that slogan leads to a false sense of security.

This fact was made very clear to me when a woman in her early fifties came into my office in tears about the thought of losing her teeth. "I've brushed my teeth twice a day and have seen my family dentist twice a year for thirty years, and at my last visit he told me that I needed full dentures because all my teeth are loose." On another occasion, in the course of a dental evaluation, I told a woman that she was in serious danger of losing all her teeth. She also broke down in tears and, when questioned, reported that her former dentist, her family dentist all her life, had told her she would lose her teeth by the time she was forty. How was I to know that her fortieth birthday was one week away?

Today, thirty years later, these women still have most of the teeth they had at that time. I also have had similar experiences with many men concerned about the prospect of dentures, but without the tears and, hence, less dramatic. The credit for their success in avoiding dentures belongs to these dedicated patients and to the great advances in dental science over these years.

Unfortunately, variations on this theme are more common than we realize. Many people brush their teeth regularly but still do not maintain a clean, odorless mouth. In order to be successful in your efforts to retain your natural teeth you must learn how to maintain excellent oral hygiene and to keep your natural teeth in a good state of repair. This usually requires the help of a caring, competent dentist.

The body does not repair worn teeth as it does other tissues. Even though dental enamel is second only to diamond in hardness, chewing eventually wears through it to expose the dentin, which is softer. The teeth become sensitive to cold, sweets, and acids; not exactly sensations sought after to enhance the pleasure of eating. No matter how lucky you may be with your inheritance of good teeth, they are affected by daily wear and tear, exposed to caustic chemicals in many foods and drugs, and bathed in saliva, an ideal culture for hundreds of bacterial strains. The stresses of life and normal use eventually take their toll. But there is hope. Proper dental care, beginning early in life, should enable you to keep your teeth for your lifetime!

There are four conditions that are common dental problems.

1. Dental caries (tooth decay); most prevalent among children, teenagers, and elderly.
2. Periodontal disease (gum disease); related primarily to oral hygiene, it affects people of all ages.
3. Erosion; a wearing away of tooth structures at the gum line.
4. Abrasion; wear on the chewing surfaces that flattens the teeth and reduces their chewing efficiency. Abrasion may also occur at the gum line from improper brushing or abrasive toothpaste.

Dental caries and periodontal disease are the result of complex bacterial processes. Both are controllable and in many cases preventable using the dental, nutritional, and biochemical knowledge now available.

Dental erosion and dental abrasion are physiochemical and mechanical processes unrelated to bacterial activity. Their slow, relentless progression makes them less preventable and actually unavoidable with advancing age. But, both conditions are treatable using current dental knowledge.

In the worst case, where some teeth are lost

despite the best efforts to keep them (accidents, lack of information, inadequate treatment, severe genetic impairment, etc.), dental implants and prostheses are now available that can do much to restore natural appearance and function.

The human body is a very complex mechanism and every individual, except identical twins, has a different set of genes. It is a mistake to assume that because something happened to a friend or someone else that it will happen to you. Despite all surface indications that make your situation seem like someone else's, the outcome can be different. Much depends on you; your attitude, your commitment, your motivation, and, of course, your genes. Finding a caring, competent dentist who will counsel and advise you and treat problems as they arise is also up to you. No one can impose or force good health on someone else. It's a strictly personal responsibility.

This book is intended to serve as your guide to teeth for a lifetime. Of course, you can't be sure you've had your teeth for your lifetime until after you're dead. But, it is reassuring to know that you have the necessary information and ability to retain the use of your natural teeth for as long as you'll need them. ✤

Chapter 1

WHO CARES?

We all have our own set of values. What is important to one person is trivial to another. This is true as much for dentists as it is for patients. We have individual goals, standards of conduct, and rules of ethics that guide our lives. Not all people really care about their personal health. Not all doctors are caring ministers of health. Many people smoke, drink to excess, use drugs, abuse their bodies, and disregard the established rules for health. It is obvious that their conduct is not conducive to good health. When ill, all their pleas for a doctor to save them are in vain, and no amount of money can buy health as long as they persist in their unhealthy lifestyles.

People who really want to enjoy good health—in dentistry that means retain their teeth for their lifetime—must live by the rules of good health and keep alert to the ever-changing environment that influences their health. For whatever reason (of birth, inheritance, or life circumstances), if they put other values before health, they pay a price. No matter how strong their inheritance, or how vigorous their appearance, nature eventually exacts its toll.

Where do you fit into this picture? Of course, you are health-motivated; why else would you be reading this? How did you get that way? How do we become what we are?

Every kid in school is expected to learn elementary arithmetic and to learn that the whole is the sum of its parts. But, who teaches a child to generalize this axiom to understand that each individual is the sum of all the positive factors minus all the negative factors that influence each of us from the time of conception, and even before. No clearer example of this effect can be demonstrated than the mothers addicted to cocaine who give birth to defective, addicted babies.

Beginning at conception we are all programmed by our genetic makeup (our heredity) over which we have no control. We grow up learning from parents, friends and teachers, and everyday experiences. Many studies have shown that by the third year of infancy, lifetime personality traits have been established. At school we learn to read newspapers, magazines, and books; at home we see commercials on television and hear them on radio. We are bombarded with information—some truth and much myth. The attitudes that we develop toward the rules of health are a very important part of our education. We must learn to separate truth from myth, to prevent illness rather than await the need for treatment, and to seek competent medical advice in an information quagmire that provides a screen for many snake oil merchants.

To summarize, our health is affected by the balance between ignorance and knowledge, misinformation and facts. We are born ignorant; it's what we learn that counts. And we can learn to value our health. We can learn to care about it. We can learn to seek the help of others who care. If it is within you to take charge of your health, you will. No one can do it for you, but caring doctors and friends can help. ✣

Chapter 2

A DENTAL LONGEVITY TEST

Given your heredity (you didn't ask for it), what do you have going, for or against you, to keep your teeth for your lifetime? Take the following test, add up the score, and we will discuss your chances. Remember, no matter what the score, modern dentistry can help you achieve that goal.

Keep score on a separate sheet of paper with two columns, one headed YES, the other NO. Check the appropriate column with your answer as you enter the number of each question. We'll total the score at the end.

1. Did your parents and grandparents have some (rarely all) of their natural teeth for their lifetime?

Answer only if you know.

a. Father
b. Mother
c. Maternal Grandfather
d. Maternal Grandmother
e. Paternal Grandfather
f. Paternal Grandmother

2. Did you have dental decay in your deciduous (baby) teeth?

3. Did you have any tooth decay as a teenager?

4. Did you have decay in your back teeth as a teenager?

5. Did you have decay in your back and front teeth as a teenager?

6. Did you have crooked teeth or need orthodontia (braces)?

7. Did you have them straightened?

8. Did you have any teeth extracted because of decay, toothache, or an accident? Don't count 3rd molars (wisdom teeth) and any extractions required for orthodontia.

9. If yes, were the missing teeth replaced?

10. Was root-canal therapy ever recommended?

11. If yes, did you have any root-canal fillings?

12. Do you smoke or chew tobacco?

13. Do you regularly eat or drink between meals any of the following?

a. Sweetened or carbonated soft drinks
b. Candy or chocolates
c. Ice Cream
d. Pie
e. Sugared cereals

f. Cake
g. Cookies
h. Other snacks

14. Do your gums bleed when you brush your teeth?

15. Do you brush your teeth *thoroughly* at least once a day?

16. Do you get a dental checkup at least once a year?

17. Is calculus formation on your teeth a problem? (Calculus is the stuff that hardens at the gum line, most commonly on the inner surface of the lower front teeth.)

18. When you bring your upper and lower teeth together and push back gently on your chin, do all your teeth meet evenly?

19. Do you have a habit of grinding your teeth?

20. Do you consider your teeth important to your general health?

21. Do you consider your smile important to your appearance?

To total your score, give yourself ten points for each correct answer

YES: 1a, b, c, d, e, f, 7, 9, 11, 15, 16, 18, 20, 21.
NO: 2, 3, 4, 5, 6, 8, 10, 12, 13a, b, c, d, e, f, g, h, 14, 17, 19.

If your score is 250 or more, without fudging, you are one of the fortunate people with good-to-excellent dentition. You should be able to retain your teeth for your lifetime in your present lifestyle. A regular dental checkup at least once a year is your best assurance that this level of dental health will be maintained. If your score is less than 250, some moderate changes should be considered along with a thorough dental diagnosis and any necessary treatment by a competent dentist. If less than 150, you are definitely at risk for false teeth and should consider seriously whether or not you are motivated to keep your teeth for your lifetime.

Since most people in the 250 category and below require the help of a competent dentist, the next question is, how do you judge competence? I'll discuss this topic later in HOW TO CHOOSE YOUR DENTIST. (Chapter 12)

The purpose of this test is to give you an idea of the role you must play if you are to keep your teeth for your lifetime. Your dentist can help; but the primary responsibility is yours—a fact many people refuse to accept. Dental science has made it possible for you to beat the rap of full dentures, no matter what your dental longevity score, if you choose to make the effort. ✤

A TOOTH AND ITS SUPPORTING TISSUES
Normal Appearance
In Cross Section

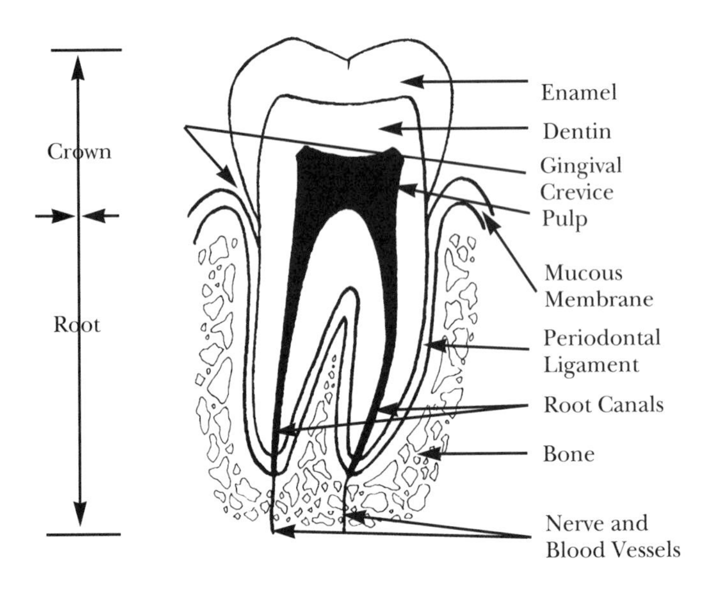

Figure 1

Chapter 3

ORAL HYGIENE IS NUMBER ONE

Oral hygiene is listed first because it is **THE** most important requirement for teeth for your lifetime. No matter what else you do, or how much money you spend to do it in an effort to keep your teeth, the long-term result depends on your ability to maintain excellent oral hygiene every day. Saying, "I brush my teeth two or three times a day" does not prove that you practice good oral hygiene.

Oral hygiene has to do with cleanliness. What is clean to one person is filth to another. Ask any housekeeper or launderer. If I sweep the floor or vacuum a carpet but don't clean in the cracks, there is plenty of stuff left to feed ants and cockroaches. In the mouth these bugs are called bacteria.

The spaces between gums and teeth are called the gingival crevice (Fig. 2). They are home for over 400 different kinds of bacteria, even in clean mouths. These bacteria form a thick, sticky film called *plaque* that adheres to the teeth like glue.

GINGIVAL CREVICE

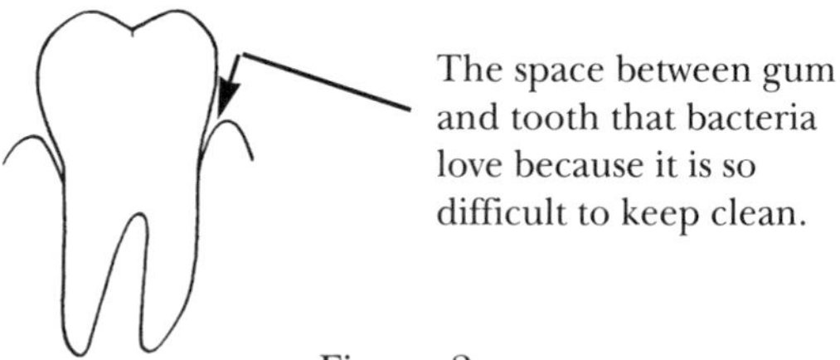

Figure 2

The deep crevices that some people have on their tongues are also great places for culturing bacteria. What we see, and usually brush, are the smooth, easy-to-reach areas of the teeth and gums.

Just as a man sweeping a carpet (according to my wife) does a half-baked job by cleaning only what he can see and reach without much effort, most people brush their teeth and gums in a la-di-da fashion and call it oral hygiene. Some who want to be really conscientious do it four or five times a day, or after every meal, but never thoroughly.

The difficulty of maintaining a clean mouth varies with the following:

- **AGE:** Children's teeth and gums are much easier to keep clean than adults'.
- **DIET:** Lots of sticky foods cling to the teeth as dental plaque that is difficult to remove, especially with frequent snacks and junk foods. Bacteria thrive on them.
- **CLEANLINESS:** Oral hygiene in adults is usually geared to their general personal hygiene. But problems arise in the mouth that may make oral hygiene much more demanding, and more difficult, for some people.
- **LONGEVITY:** Aging creates larger spaces

between the teeth and increases the difficulty of cleaning them at a time when vision, coordination, and motivation also may be on the decline. This often leads to greater dental problems after age 65. Older people have to work harder on all aspects of personal hygiene to look as atttractive as they were in their youth.

- **PERIODONTAL DISEASE:** The spaces between the teeth also become more open as a result of periodontal disease, which may occur at any age. Keeping these areas clean and free of infection becomes more difficult as the disease progresses. Dental researchers report that 80% to 95% of the United States population has periodontal disease. It is a national health problem that does not get media attention because it is not life-threatening. What *is* being done about it is discussed more fully below.
- **DEXTERITY:** People vary in their abilities to use their hands and manipulate tools. As in tennis, where you take lessons from a tennis pro to improve your skill with a racket, in oral hygiene you consult an oral-hygiene pro, your dental hygienist, to become skillful in maintaining a clean mouth.
- **MEDICATIONS:** Prolonged use of antibiotics may alter the bacterial environment in your mouth and result in a fungus infection. It usually appears as a thick white coating on the tongue that can be removed with vigorous brushing.

When we consider all the things that influence oral hygiene, it is not surprising that these problems affect 90% of the population at some time of life. The fact that periodontal disease is a chronic, low-grade infection, often undiagnosed, should make it clear that it is wise to learn good oral-hygiene habits early and to pay increasing attention to them as you get older. In order to succeed at this, most people need instruction from their dentist or dental hygienist along with periodic checkups. Depending on the schools they attended or their personal preferences, these professionals in oral hygiene may vary in their recommended toothbrushing techniques. Or, they may have specific instructions tailored to the need of the individual patient. There is no wrong or right road to oral hygiene; whatever works for you to achieve the goal, a clean mouth, without injury to the oral tissues, is correct for you.

An effective oral-hygiene program usually requires five steps, not necessarily in this order.

1. An antibacterial mouth rinse, preferably with fluoride.
2. A toothpick to wipe away the plaque in the narrow gingival crevice, one tooth at a time. (Fig. 3).

TOOTHPICK TECHNIQUE

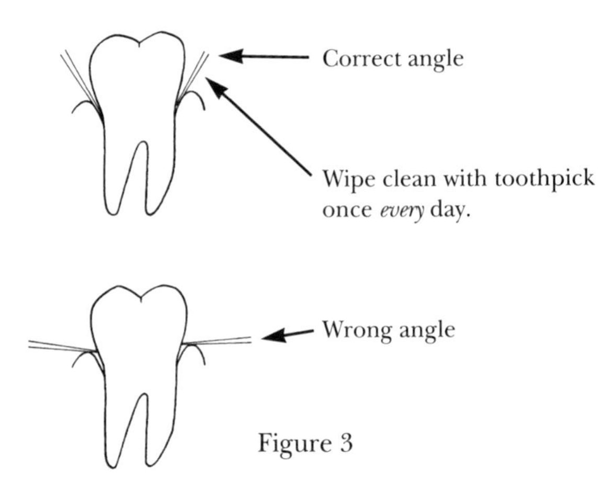

Figure 3

Some people accept the routine of gingival massage with a toothpick more readily and get better results by combining this with a pleasurable procedure such as watching television, bathing, showering, or driving.

3. Dental floss to remove plaque and debris from between the teeth where the toothbrush cannot reach. A four-inch loop is easier to hold and helps avoid snapping the floss onto the gums. (Figs. 4ab and 5)

INCORRECT TECHNIQUE

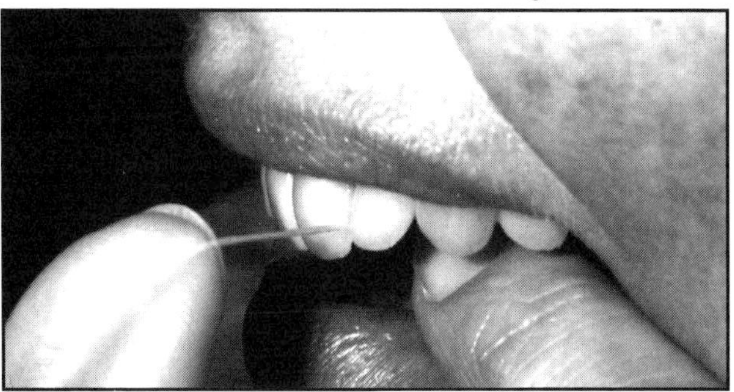

When the floss snaps through the contact, it strikes the gum, causing pain and bleeding.

Figure 4a

CORRECT TECHNIQUE

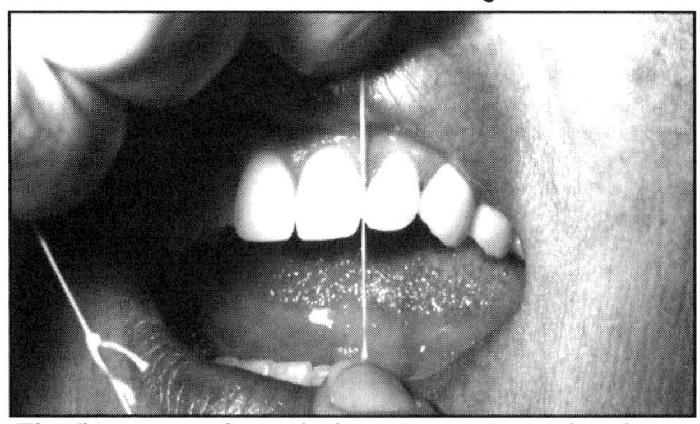

The floss passes through the contact. It can then be redirected to wipe the adjacent surfaces up and down.

Figure 4b

DENTAL FLOSS LOOP

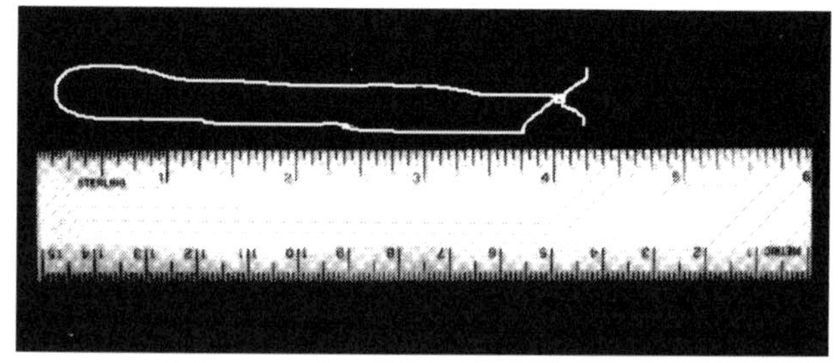

A loop of dental floss is easier to use.

Figure 5

4. A toothbrush and non-abrasive, fluoride toothpaste to clean the easy-to-reach surfaces of the teeth and remove debris and dead cells from the adjacent gums, cheeks, and tongue. The practice of some people who prefer a brush with stiff bristles to "scrub" the teeth and a more abrasive toothpaste for its whitening effect often causes severe abrasion and premature loss of enamel. A battery -powered toothbrush now available provides a soft bristle and rotary motion to reach all areas of the mouth effectively without "scrubbing." When used with a mildly abrasive toothpaste (all toothpastes and powders depend on abrasive action for their effectiveness), this toothbrush helps achieve good oral hygiene without injury to the enamel or soft tissues.
5. Thorough rinsing to remove all the loosened material. This requires vigorous use of cheeks and tongue to force water between and around all the teeth. For those incapable of this, power driven oral irrigators are available.

It should be obvious that good oral hygiene is not a two-minute procedure. And, as stated above, it should be learned from an oral-hygiene pro, your dentist or dental hygienist.

Toothbrushes, toothpastes, dental floss, and toothpicks come in a bewildering variety of sizes, shapes, and formulations. The American Dental Association provides the dental public with an ongoing program that evaluates and rates these products for safety and effectiveness, based on reliable scientific data. The Seal of Approval of the ADA is your assurance that you may use the product without danger to your health (See Appendix A).

If you follow a thorough dental-hygiene routine at least once a day (it will take five to ten minutes each time until you become experienced), you will be practicing good dental hygiene. Most people prefer to clean their mouths at night before retiring and again in the morning—an excellent routine as long as the job is done thoroughly both times. Those who are most meticulous brush mornings, evenings, and after meals.

If you are under the regular supervision of your dentist and/or dental hygienist, you should get good grades at check-up time. If not, they will let you know why.

The Dental Hygiene Toolbox

New devices are continually appearing in the marketplace and are advertised as the secret to good oral hygiene. Buyer beware! The effectiveness of any oral-hygiene device depends on the skill and motivation of the person behind it—on a daily basis, and that person is you. Some tools have limited usefulness where there are special problems of dexterity or coordination; in the physically handicapped, retarded, and senile, for example. They are most helpful when used in the basic program just outlined.

To be specific, a powered water spray is helpful for effective rinsing, but it does not remove plaque and is not a substitute for the toothpick, toothbrush, and dental floss.

Power-driven toothbrushes are helpful and, in some cases, indispensable. However, they do not remove plaque any more thoroughly than the pick, brush, and floss combination; and like any other oral hygiene procedure, their effectiveness depends on instruction from your dentist or dental hygienist. As mentioned above, the rotary, soft-bristle brush facilitates plaque removal for many people and enables even the handicapped to reach all areas of the mouth.

Plaque-prevention toothpastes may help retard plaque formation and are therefore useful for everyone, but they do not remove plaque once it is formed. (It builds up daily and, in some mouths, rapidly.)

Tooth-whiteners in paste or powder form intended to bleach teeth may be misleading. Once all the stains are removed from tooth enamel, usually with a mild abrasive, the natural color of the tooth, which is what you see, cannot be changed without chemical bleaching. You are looking at the internal color of the tooth (dentin) shining through the translucent enamel.

Individual teeth may become discolored by internal bleeding as the result of a blow or an accident because the tiny blood vessels in the pulp are ruptured. Bleaching such a tooth is a dental procedure that involves root-canal therapy and chemical treatment of the tooth from within. It is most successful when done promptly after the injury. The best way to change tooth color is with baked porcelain bonded veneers (See Chapter 11, Cosmetic Dentistry.).

Bad Breath Phobia

No discussion of oral hygiene would be complete without some comment about halitosis. The fear of "bad breath," the social stigma that it carries, and the fact that the offender may be totally unaware of it are the strongest motivation for some people to keep their mouths clean. How can you be sure about it?

Be thorough in carrying out your daily oral-hygiene routine! The most common cause of halitosis is periodontal disease associated with inadequate oral hygiene. To be doubly sure, make an agreement with someone close to you to let you know if your breath is offensive in exchange for providing the same service.

Be aware that a dry mouth increases the tendency to have bad breath. The stress and tension people feel at social functions may create dry-mouth halitosis at a time when they are most anxious to avoid it. A peppermint lozenge that helps keep your saliva flowing may be a lifesaver under these conditions. If halitosis persists despite your best efforts to control it, you should consult your dentist; there may be oral infections that must be treated or some systemic disease that requires the attention of your medical doctor.

The fact that halitosis is socially unacceptable is reason enough to make oral hygiene a Number One concern. But the most important reasons for giving oral hygiene your highest priority, if you want to keep your teeth for your lifetime, may be stated simply: **Clean only those teeth that you want to keep.**

In the current, nationwide drive to control the costs of health care, it seems obvious that prevention of disease should be the primary goal. Periodontal disease is preventable. Accordingly, the American Dental Association has launched a nationwide campaign to focus the attention of dentists on the need to emphasize oral hygiene to their patients in a systematic, sustained educational program. At the same time, a major educational effort will be directed through the media to inform the public of this insidious and widespread national health problem. The emphasis will be on the major health benefits and reduced dental expenses that can be achieved with the prevenion of periodontal disease.

That message, briefly stated, is that if you want teeth for your lifetime, **make oral hygiene your Number One dental concern.** ✜

Chapter 4

CROOKED TEETH

To some people, their appearance is like a movie set—as long as the front looks good, it doesn't matter what's in back; that part is not seen by the audience. Others keep their cars painted and polished and neglect the motor and transmission until they are stranded. When applied to teeth, this attitude can lead to dentures.

How teeth function is just as important as their appearance in maintaining good dental health. The front and back teeth must be aligned in their proper functional relationship when a dentist straightens crooked teeth. I have seen dentists advertise the straightening of the six upper and six lower front teeth at bargain rates. To a Hollywood-type who thinks teeth are a movie set (all you see is what's up front), this may be attractive, but it is not likely to provide teeth for a lifetime. Certainly cosmetics are an important part of dentistry, and new bonding materials have greatly improved cosmetic procedures. They get better all the time, and it is a challenge to dentists to keep up with the changes.

However, to neglect tooth function and concentrate on cosmetics only is a common and serious error for the long term. Nevertheless, some dentists feel compelled to do so in their efforts to please their patients. The goal should be good function along with ideal appearance. The way teeth work in chewing and swallowing has much to do with how long they will last. When properly aligned, teeth look better, they are easier to clean (which helps avoid periodontal disease), they do a better job of chewing (helping to avoid digestion problems), and they don't wear out as fast.

Fortunately, if you don't like the appearance of your smile, there's a good chance you can do something about it that will improve all your teeth and help you avoid dentures. Modern dentistry usually makes it possible to move teeth at any age; to line them up as perfectly as you would like them to be; to change their color, shape, and size; to realign the jaws, if necessary, and to change the appearance of the face.

For all these reasons, if your teeth are crooked or unattractive, it is wise to consult your dentist about the best way to align them for better appearance and normal function. The problem may be minor and treatable by your family dentist, or you may need to see an orthodontist who specializes in straightening teeth. In any case, no treatment should be started without a thorough diagnosis. If the problem is severe, it may be necessary to consult an oral surgeon to reposition the jaws or even create a chin; a speech therapist to correct bad swallowing patterns or tongue habits; or a periodontist if there are problems in that area. Your family dentist should guide you through all of this. A correct diagnosis, in advance, is the most important part of all dental procedures. If you have doubts, don't hesitate to get a second opinion. No matter how crooked your teeth are, or hopeless their appearance, treatment by competent dentists regularly produce remarkable improvements. ✜

Chapter 5

PAINFUL TEETH

A toothache, like a nail in your shoe, can become extremely painful. Unlike the nail, which you would remove immediately if you wanted to walk, the toothache may go away within minutes and be forgotten. When the toothache returns, as it usually does, the pain lasts a little longer, eventually feeling like a nail in your head.

Dental pain is a warning sign that says, "See your dentist." Each time the pain returns, the warning is repeated. Despite this protective shield provided by nature, many people ignore the warning(s) until the problem becomes a genuine crisis. If it occurs in the middle of the night or on a holiday weekend or during your vacation when your dentist is not available, the experience can be unforgettably unpleasant. It often results in the loss of the offending tooth or teeth. Some people get so distraught that they have all their teeth removed in order to be sure they will have no more toothaches. Unfortunately, this action brings on the much more serious problems of living with false teeth for the rest of your life. If you understand the progression of dental pain, it may help you avoid this normally avoidable mistake.

Sensitivity to cold is usually the first sign of a problem tooth. Dentin that has lost its covering of protective enamel becomes increasingly sensitive to temperature changes (especially cold), to pH (acidity) changes in the saliva, and to friction. The loss of enamel, the remarkably durable and irreplaceable protective coating on teeth provided by nature, is usually due to one of the following:

- DECAY—bacterial and chemical activity have destroyed the enamel surface and the process has invaded the unprotected dentin. The enamel disintegration usually begins between adjacent teeth where it is hard to keep the teeth clean or in the deep grooves on the chewing surfaces (Fig. 6).

DENTAL DECAY (CARIES)

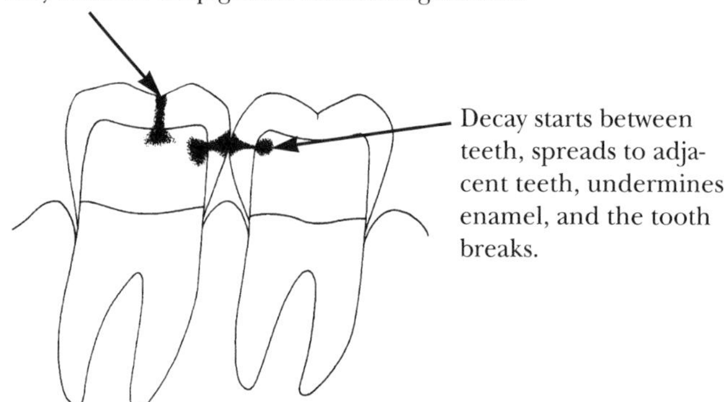

Figure 6

• EROSION—slow, chemical removal of enamel that exposes dentin. This usually occurs at the gum line (Fig. 7).

• ABRASION—slow, wearing away of the enamel to expose dentin, usually on the chewing surfaces (Fig. 7).

ENAMEL EROSION AND ABRASION

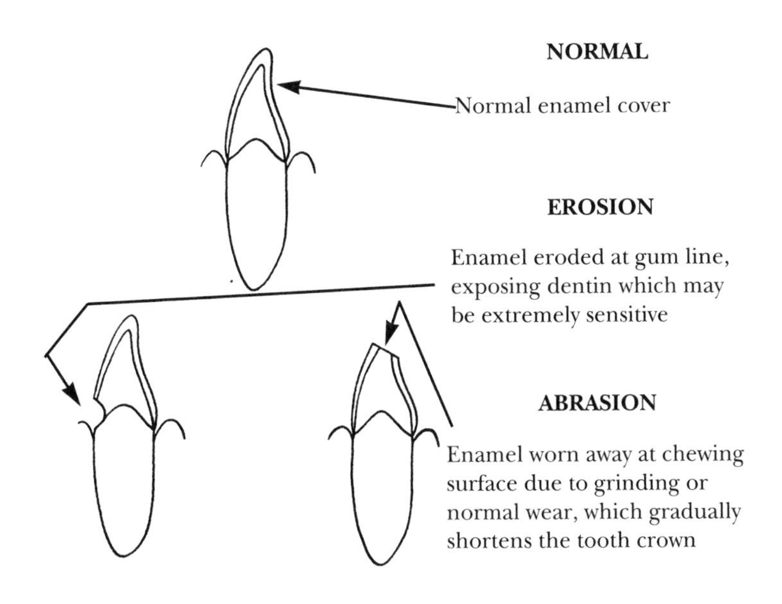

Figure 7

• FRACTURE—the result of undermining tooth decay, traumatic injury, or abnormal or excessive chewing forces.

• INFECTION—acute or chronic inflammation of the dental pulp (nerve) or periodontal (gum) tissues may cause pain that varies from mild to excruciating (the unforgettable toothache) (Fig. 8).

DENTAL PULP INFECTION

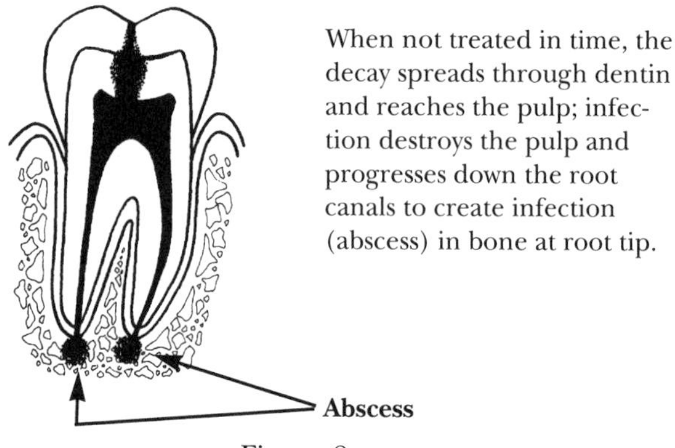

Figure 8

Treated in the early stages, all these conditions are repairable. Only decay and periodontal disease are preventable. Erosion and abrasion may not become serious until old age, when time takes its toll and these processes affect almost everyone with natural teeth.

Sensitivity to cold is usually the first warning of a sick tooth. The longer it is ignored or left untreated, the more likely that the pulp will be destroyed by infection and that root canal therapy will be needed to save the tooth. This costly procedure can usually be avoided by seeing your dentist for diagnosis and treatment promptly after the first warning pain.

Sensitivity to heat, where heat is more painful than cold, is an indication that the dental pulp is seriously impaired and that endodontic (root canal) treatment will probably be required to save the tooth.

Sensitivity to pressure is a warning that a tooth is under abnormal stress during chewing or that there is some inflammation of the pulp and/or periodontal (gum) tissues.

Fracture of teeth is a common cause of dentin exposure that requires immediate attention to protect the dental pulp.

Failure to heed the first warning (sensitivity to cold) in any of the just-described situations is frequently due to fear of dental treatment, ignorance of the consequences, or plain old neglect. It may result in having to make a choice between root canal therapy and extraction in order to eliminate the infection. In most cases, root canal therapy, despite the cost, is preferable to extraction and is less expensive in the long run. ✥

Chapter 6

JAW PAIN, JOINT PAIN, TMJ, AND TMD

Stories about excruciating dental pain are part of our folklore, handed down from generation to generation. These stories date back to the times when the only treatment for dental pain was tooth extraction, and this final act had to be done without the benefit of anaesthesia. Today our fear of dentistry is reinforced regularly by dental horror stories because, to quote an old adage, "bad news travels around the world while good news is still lacing up its boots." Occasionally we hear reports of dental pain that are genuine personal experiences. They are rare considering the millions of dental services provided daily without pain because it is controlled or eliminated entirely using modern drugs and general anaesthesia when necessary. The point here is that when it comes to preventing and relieving pain, dentists today do an outstanding job in an area where intense pain is part of folklore.

Headache is the most common complaint of pain. Just look at the variety of pain relievers advertised and sold by a billion-dollar industry, and the range of their effectiveness, from mild to knockout potential. The reason for this is that headache can have many causes (sometimes they are related), which makes its diagnosis and treatment often difficult. Among those causes, the teeth, the jaws, and the jaw joints (temporomandibular joints, or TMJ) are frequent participants. Headache is usually considered a strictly medical problem; you see your doctor. Toothache is just as clearly a dental problem; you see your dentist. Jaw pains and associated TMJ pain may be a medical/dental problem that requires the combined skills of medical and dental specialists.

For example, consider the presence of persistent, vague pain in the upper jaws in the area of the molar (back) teeth. An infection of the sinus adjacent to the teeth could be responsible for the pain, which is really a medical problem if there are no infected teeth in the area. Since the painful teeth may draw attention to the problem first, you consult the dentist whose job is to make sure there is no dental infection. If the teeth and gums are okay, you will be referred to your family doctor for diagnosis.

The overlap of medical and dental sources of pain is even more common in the area of the TMJ. These jaw joints, one on each side of your face, are the most complex joints in the body. They are also close to the distribution centers of nerves, blood vessels, and muscles that control movements and function of your head, neck, tongue, eyes, facial expression, chewing, and swallowing; including also the sensory nerves to the teeth. Unravelling the interactions in this complicated network can be a serious challenge. In cases of severe pain in this area the joints themselves may be normal, and to label the symptoms as TMJ Syndrome would be inaccurate. The correct label for all the painful conditions related to the TMJ area is Temporomandibular Disorder (TMD).

The identification of the source(s) of the pain in some cases may be extremely difficult, and may include such unsuspected factors as systemic disease, psychological and neurological problems. Reports are not uncommon of long-suffering patients who have been referred to a succession of specialists including an ear, nose, and throat specialist, a neurologist, a psychiatrist, and an oral surgeon, all in cooperation with medical and dental general practitioners. Not infrequently, the cause is entirely dental, and failure of a medical doctor to suspect the dental origin can prolong the suffering for the patient. Conversely, an overzealous dentist unaware of the medical nature of the problem also may prolong the pain unnecessarily.

While the medical label TMD is used to identify this complex pain, the actual diagnosis leading to treatment requires identification of the source or cause of the symptoms. They may vary from acute pain in the area of one or both jaw joints to a long-standing, chronic head or neck pain; from a slight clicking of the jaw joint to actual locking such that the jaw cannot be moved at all. Pain on chewing may be the result of misalignment of teeth or stress on the TMJ from other causes. Sore teeth or painful joints in the morning are usually signs of bruxism (grinding the teeth) which may occur while sleeping. Treatment may be as straightforward as adjusting the occlusion of the teeth (the way they come together in chewing) to provide proper function or complicated enough to involve maxillofacial surgery, neurosurgery, or psychotherapy. Realignment of the jaws is called orthognathic surgery.

Because the patient may be in great distress, it is sometimes necessary to resort to immediate pain-relieving treatment before the diagnosis is confirmed. A common practice is to construct a plastic device worn in the patient's mouth to neutralize stress to the joints that may be caused by malocclusion. Relief from pain is sometimes dramatic, indicating that the malocclusion was indeed the source of the problem. Whatever the benefits of this device (an occlusal guard or occlusion deprogrammer), it is only a diagnostic tool and is worn only temporarily until more definite treatment is completed. This also allows time to obtain a second opinion where surgery or elaborate treatment is recommended. The primary role of the dentist in these cases is to rule out the teeth, especially the occlusion, as a possible source of the problem. ✣

Chapter 7

MOUTH INFECTIONS

Infections of the mouth can affect teeth, gums, and bone, singly or together. In Chapter 3, while discussing oral hygiene, I referred to the fact that more than 400 different microorganisms may call the mouth their home. Dental decay and periodontal disease were discussed as the two most common effects of those invaders. Not all the bugs are harmful; some may even be beneficial. It doesn't take a genius to understand that maintaining a clean mouth, as free as possible of the disease-producing bacteria, will help prolong the life of your teeth. Cleanliness is your responsibility and you alone get the most benefits from your efforts.

But what about virus infections, many of which are airborne and may have nothing to do with your oral hygiene? Can you avoid them? The answer is no. The most you can do is reduce your risk by limiting your exposure to them. Viruses are so numerous, so pervasive, and so changeable that we really don't know they're around until it's too late and we are ill. The common cold is the best example. Much as we dislike colds, despite billions of dollars spent on research for a cure, we still cannot avoid them. To reduce the risk of catching influenza, many doctors recommend flu vaccine (shots), renewed every year to combat the current strains of flu virus. This works well for most people and is recommended especially for children and the aged. There is, however, no sure treatment for virus infections of the mouth. They appear as sores, usually referred to as ulcers, on any of the oral soft tissues; the lips, gums, cheeks, tongue, or roof of the mouth.

The fact that ulcers of the mouth have many different causes may make diagnosis difficult. Occasionally they are easy to identify, as in an irritation by a sharp tooth or ill-fitting denture. Sometimes they disappear gradually without treatment (the disease runs its course); sometimes they spread rapidly and involve large areas of the mouth and cause much discomfort. They may even become life-threatening.

When ulcers appear, painful or not, you should visit your dentist promptly. Some serious diseases such as herpes, AIDS, and oral cancer may be first identified as small ulcers in the mouth. They should not be neglected because they respond best to early treatment. The likelihood of an ulcer in your mouth being diagnosed as one of these diseases is extremely remote unless your lifestyle has put you at greater than average risk, as would be the case for cancer if you smoke cigarettes and, even worse, chew tobacco. In the case of AIDS, its connection with sexual promiscuity has been well established and thoroughly publicized.

The danger of cross-contamination between dentist and patient in the transmission of viral diseases (including hepatitis B, not mentioned under ulcers because it does not produce oral symptoms), has resulted in the adoption of rigid protective measures in most dental offices. It is now standard procedure for dentists, hygienists, and assistants to wear rubber gloves, masks, and protective eyeglasses. Instrument sterilization equipment has been improved along with higher standards of disinfection. Even trash disposal has been rerouted to avoid transmission of infectious material.

The bottom line on mouth infections is the lifestyle of the individual, his or her awareness of the environmental hazards, and the measures to control them in the dental office that are available to the dentist. The reassuring note is that 98% of all oral ulcers are self-limiting and disappear spontaneously. The bacterial infections in the mouth which are most common are dental decay, periodontal disease, and pulp infections which are readily controlled with modern dental procedures and appropriate medications. ✜

Chapter 8

MISSING TEETH

A Halloween pumpkin face carved with alternate teeth missing is always good for a laugh with kids, but it's not funny if the face is yours. Your smile has a great bearing on your self-esteem; it's important that we feel good about ourselves. That's why many people spend money willingly to replace missing front teeth, straighten them, or bond them with veneers (thin porcelain coatings) to make their smiles look good. See COSMETIC DENTISTRY (Chapter 11). But teeth must do more than look good if they are to last a lifetime.

You should replace missing teeth not only for cosmetic reasons, but also to restore normal function and distribute the chewing forces evenly among all the back teeth. The importance of this is lost to most people with limited budgets for dental repairs and who have major interest only in appearance. Unfortunately for them, cost is frequently the deciding factor in dental treatment.

The compromises made often result in maintaining the appearance of the front teeth for a few years while they become overworked, overstressed, and worn excessively because the back teeth are not contributing to normal function. These patients lose their teeth one at a time as they become unrepairable. And even with care, over a period of time and with advancing age, the entire dentition (teeth, gums, and supporting bone) gradually deteriorates, along with all the other body tissues. Soft tissues and bone, if injured or broken, are repaired by normal healing processes. But nature does not repair or restore teeth when they are decayed, fractured, eroded, or worn flat by usage. When the restoration of teeth to their normal shape and function requires treatment of the entire dentition (oral reconstruction), the cost can total thousands of dollars—a major concern for people approaching retirement. The only alternatives usually are partial or full dentures.

The most common cause of loss of teeth is periodontal disease which, if untreated, leads to the slow, progressive, and often unnoticed deterioration of the bone supporting the teeth. Typically, it is associated with inadequate oral hygiene. Other related, less-common causes are systemic bone disease such as osteoporosis, the effects of radiation therapy for treatment of oral cancer, and heavy-metal poisoning (lead, mercury, etc.).

Advanced tooth decay is generally assumed to be reason enough for extracting a tooth, but with modern dental treatment a tooth usually can be saved with root-canal therapy (endodontia) and restored to normal function with a cast metal or baked porcelain crown. Of course, this is costly; the price of dental neglect. It could probably have been avoided with early treatment at the first warning symptom; usually sensitivity to cold.

It is wrong to blame patient neglect for all missing teeth, however. Accidents involving the face can cause teeth to be evulsed (knocked out), fractured, or dislodged in such a way that repair is impossible. Genetic defects cause teeth to be missing because they never developed; this problem is often traceable through various members of a family and through successive generations. The only exception to the importance of replacing missing teeth are third molars (wisdom teeth). They may be genetically missing or, if present, malpositioned or impacted (growing horizontally) in bone so that they must be removed to avoid or relieve complications. The stories you hear about wisdom-tooth extractions make this procedure scary to anyone faced with it. Even though the surgery is usually done under general anaesthesia and is painless, the post-operative pain characteristic of all bone surgery is unpredictable. At best, it is minor and easily controlled with mild pain relievers. At the other extreme, it may be difficult to control even with strong drugs and may result in an extended (two-week) period of painful recovery.

Replacement of missing teeth is a routine procedure in dentistry and many general dentists become very skillful in this area of treatment. Dental restorations are made with a variety of materials used as fillings, veneers, and partial or full crowns. Scientists using modern technology are continually improving the quality and appearance of these materials, but for the chewing surfaces of the teeth, where the greatest forces are exerted, nothing exceeds cast gold for durability and comfort. For aesthetics, baked porcelain is still the preferred choice because it is unaffected by mouth fluids and the foods we eat.

IMPORTANCE OF REPLACING MISSING TEETH

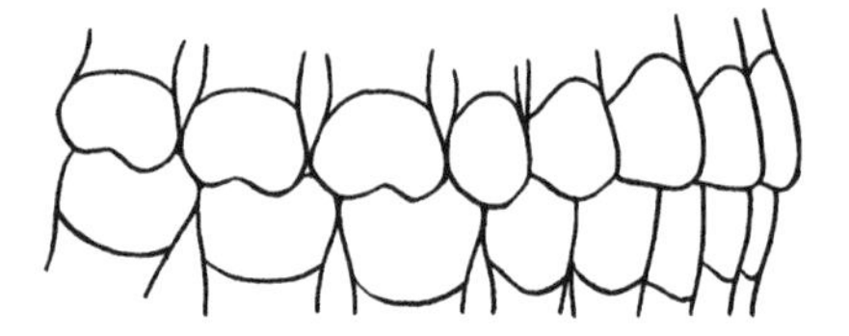

In normal occlusion, chewing teeth are in proper relation for normal function.

Progressive problems that result when an extracted lower molar is not replaced. Teeth move, causing:

Open contacts—spaces between teeth
Malfunction—chewing interferences
Cavities due to food impaction
Periodontal disease due to food impaction

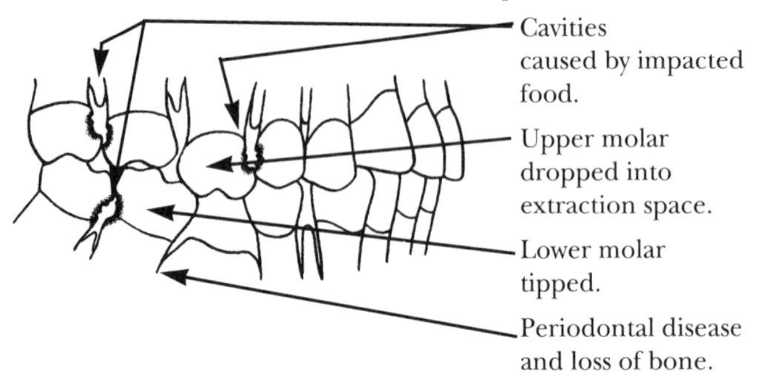

Fixed prosthesis (fixed bridge) restores normal function.

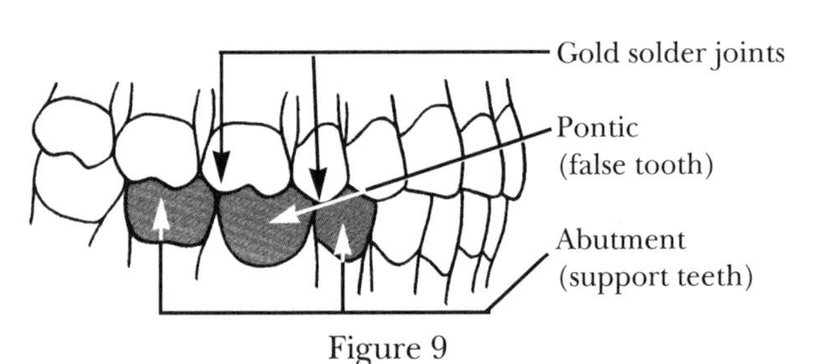

Figure 9

Complicated cases involving all or most of the teeth in oral reconstruction are sometimes referred to a specialist (prosthodontist) who is better equipped by training and experience to meet the special needs of these patients.

In summary, teeth should be replaced soon after they are extracted in order to preserve the dental arch and prevent the remaining teeth from "drifting." When this is allowed to happen, the teeth move out of place and spaces open between them. Food impaction then makes them difficult to keep clean. The periodontal infection that follows may result in the additional loss of teeth, one or two at a time.

The restorations needed to replace missing teeth or close spaces between them should be completed when recommended by your dentist, or, if there is reason for delay, as soon as practical. ✣

Chapter 9

DENTAL PROSTHESES AND DENTURES

Canes, crutches, and walkers are a great help to people having difficulty walking or maintaining their balance. Eyeglasses help people to see better and protect their eyes from flying debris. But what about those who lose a leg or an arm or become blind? Artificial arms and legs are useful substitutes for lost limbs; functional artificial eyes are still only a fantasy. In any case, these substitutes for natural body parts (prosthes*is* is one, prosthes*es* if more than one) are a great improvement over the conditions that would exist without them.

When just one tooth is lost, the dentition is impaired, and there is a loss of normal function. As each additional tooth is lost, chewing becomes increasingly difficult. Missing teeth can be replaced to fill in the spaces between the remaining natural teeth and restore normal function. Replacement teeth may be cemented permanently to the remaining natural teeth (a fixed prosthesis or "bridge") or they may be removable (a partial denture or removable prosthesis). If all the teeth are lost, dental implants may be used to serve as anchors to attach the prosthesis to the jaw. This technology is a recent advance in dental science. Without implants, full dentures are referred to as false teeth. The negative attitude toward full dentures is often expressed by the saying, "Be true to your teeth or they will be false to you." But, as in the case of artificial limbs, false teeth are a welcome substitute for no teeth at all.

The thrust of this book is to help you avoid dental prostheses of any kind; to keep your natural teeth functioning for your lifetime. But lack of information, neglect, accidents, and, unfortunately, poor dentistry, are among the many reasons that cause most people to lose some teeth in their lifetime. When that happens, choices must be made. This is when you need the help of a caring family dentist. Since each individual case must be decided on its own merits, there is no substitute for the informed judgment of a competent dentist. And because expense is often the controlling factor, indecision may lead to neglect, and over a period of time the problems worsen, costs can increase, and more teeth are lost. This is the sad road to full dentures.

Here is some information to serve as a guide to help you avoid full dentures. Depending on the number and location of missing teeth, the following restorations should be completed when recommended by your dentist.

For single-tooth restorations, a fixed (cemented) prosthesis is usually preferable. This is often referred to as a fixed bridge (Fig. 10).

FIXED BRIDGE

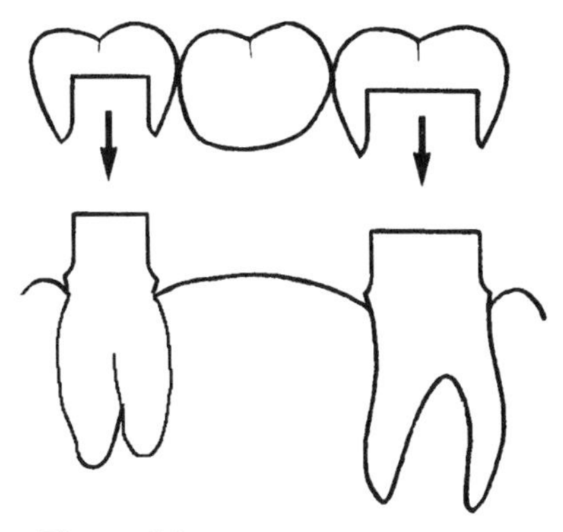

Figure 10

Multiple-tooth restorations depend on the presence of natural teeth for their support and may be fixed or removable, depending on the arrangement of the natural teeth and those to be replaced. Fixed restorations are usually the preferred choice; they feel and look more natural, they are more comfortable in chewing, and in the presence of good oral hygiene, more long-lasting. But, they are more costly.

Dental implants are becoming more reliable as anchors for fixed and removable prostheses, from a single tooth to multiple restorations and full dentures. Unlike dentures, which rest on the mucous membranes (gums) that cover the jaw bone where teeth are missing, implants are anchored in the underlying bone and give the patient the feel of natural teeth. Their use is limited in two ways: Not all jaw bone is dense enough to support them—a CAT scan of the jaw is usually part of the diagnostic procedure—and their cost is often a financial deterrent.

All prosthetic restorations in the mouth increase the need for meticulous oral hygiene while they compound the difficulty of maintaining it. The most common cause of failure of dental prostheses, fixed and removable, is plaque formation and the associated bacterial infections around the supporting teeth (abutments).

Cleaning under fixed bridges and around abutment teeth can be more difficult than with natural teeth; and the problems become worse with age, as mentioned in the discussion of oral hygiene in Chapter 3.

Full dentures are not the end of dental problems that some people imagine them to be. As bony support is lost and the mouth changes over a period of time, the dentures become painful, loose, ill-fitting, and require periodic relining. In order to prevent a collapsed appearance of the face, the dentures should be remade at least every ten years at a not-insignificant expense. The need for adjustments to relieve sore spots in the mouth varies greatly among denture wearers, but all are familiar with this chronic source of discomfort. And the ability to chew with dentures also varies greatly; some people do surprisingly well, and others have great difficulty learning to use them. Some never do. A very small fraction become so disturbed psychologically that they end up in mental hospitals. Lastly, it takes a skilled dentist and a cooperative patient to make dentures look so much like natural teeth that your friends don't know you have them.

The encouraging word about dental prostheses, and to a lesser extent full dentures, is that they can be extremely effective in restoring function and prolonging the life of the dentition. A fringe benefit is the prolonged life of the patient. To the patient, the cosmetic value often is most important as a source of restored self-esteem, self-confidence, and projected image. ✣

Chapter 10

WORN-OUT TEETH

Horses, cows, rabbits, and many other animals have teeth that never stop growing. Their diet is coarse vegetation, including lots of sand, which would cause the chewing surfaces to wear flat to the gums in a few years if their teeth did not grow at a slow, continuous rate. Obviously, we are not herbivorous animals.

Humans eat meat and vegetables; we are omnivorous, and our teeth are designed to eat all forms of food (preferably without any sand). Given a life span of about sixty years, our teeth, though worn flat and inefficient for chewing, would last as long as we needed them; provided, of course, that dental decay or periodontal problems did not intervene. However, our increasing life span (80 to 90 years) creates dental problems not provided for by Mother Nature. Modern dental care enables many people to reach age 65 with most of their teeth still intact and functioning. But those many years of chewing three meals a day will have flattened the once-pointed chewing surfaces (cusps), and gallons of coffee, tea, fruit juices, salad dressings, and wine that have flowed over them will have stained, discolored, and eroded all the teeth in characteristic patterns. All of this usually progresses at a slow rate without any discomfort to the individual. The teeth may survive this slow deterioration until age 80 or 90 (there are people with teeth to prove it) but in the great majority of cases, pain, discomfort, or vanity dictates a visit to the dentist. Here's why: Dental enamel becomes more brittle with age and teeth fracture more easily. This is more common in the molars and premolars (bicuspids). Badly eroded teeth become so worn away at the gum line that they may break under excessive chewing stress, leaving only the root and a painful exposed nerve. This occurs more frequently with front teeth and creates a dental emergency requiring the immediate attention of your dentist.

Aging also affects the bone supporting the teeth, as it does with all the other bony structures of the body. As bone is lost around the teeth, the gums recede and give the appearance of being "long in the tooth." The effects of this process can be serious. Spaces between the teeth enlarge and become more difficult to keep clean. Trapped food provides a perfect breeding place for the bacterial processes of tooth decay and periodontal disease. In the absence of meticulous daily oral hygiene, gums become swollen and inflamed, occasionally painful, and chronically infected. They bleed easily. Their odor can be exceedingly offensive—persistent "bad breath." No mouthwash masks it for long. The end result is advanced periodontal disease that usually requires the services of a dental specialist (periodontist). The root surfaces uncovered in the course of treatment are not protected with enamel and are even more susceptible to decay (Fig. 11).

PROGRESSIVE BONE LOSS FROM PERIODONTAL DISEASE

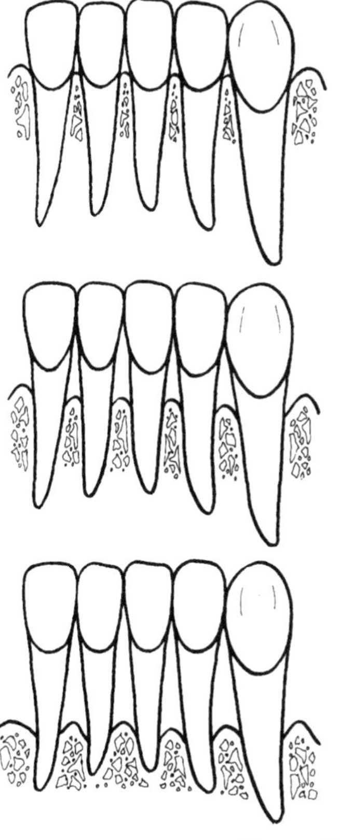

Normal Bony Support fills spaces between roots.

Progressive Loss of Bony Support causes spaces between teeth to increase and makes them difficult to clean. The resulting infection speeds up the loss of bone.

Advanced Periodontal Disease. Bony support almost all gone—not repairable—teeth become loose and gums infected.

Figure 11

All of this goes on as we get older; what is different among us is the rate of progression. *Thoroughness in daily oral hygiene slows it down!* There is no way of reversing this process any more than we can restore youth to aching bones and muscles. Dentists can help retard the progress of this deterioration and, as in other areas of medicine, restore the appearance of youth. But success in this effort is limited by at least two important factors.

First is the recognition that teeth do not function in a vacuum. They are part of a complex mechanism for chewing, swallowing, and talking with many interrelated components. The jaw joints are the most complicated joints in the body, and their complex motions are driven by powerful muscles. Biting pressures can be hundreds of pounds and any misalignment of teeth or jaws can be very destructive. Fortunately, our mouths learn to adjust to minor misalignments and avoid or defer major damage. The treatment of individual teeth as they decay, fracture, or are lost due to accident, infection, or periodontal disease serves the needs of dental patients until the time when the entire dentition is in need of repairs—usually due to age. We may compare the dentition to an automobile engine which we tune up, changing oil and spark plugs regularly until the time comes when we must completely rebuild it or exchange it for a new one. Unlike the new engine, which is as good as the one it replaces when it was new, old teeth cannot be exchanged for new ones that look and feel like the original dentition. When the dentition is worn out, usually by the age of sixty, the alternatives may be (1) complete reconstruction with gold and porcelain crowns, (2) dentures, or (3) dental implants.

Complete reconstruction of natural teeth usually involves 28 units (32 if all four wisdom teeth are present) because every missing tooth must be replaced or rebuilt along with the remaining natural teeth. This is a job that cannot be done piecemeal, as most dentistry is done. It is referred to as oral reconstruction and may require the skill and knowledge of a dentist with special training, a prosthodontist.

Dentures, unlike the new engine which restores excellent performance, are at best only one-third as efficient as natural teeth.

Implants have been used by dentists for about 25 years with limited success. Intense dental research and improvements in materials and techniques have made implants today a recommended procedure in carefully selected cases. Their use is limited, and cost is frequently a deterrent. But they come closer than any alternative prosthesis to restoring the feel of natural teeth.

This leads to the second problem with worn-out teeth; the cost of repairing all of them at the same time. It varies greatly depending on the condition and number of the remaining natural teeth; the need for periodontal therapy (gum treatment), endodontic therapy (root-canal treatment), tooth alignment (orthodontia), and jaw alignment (orthognathic surgery). If all these specialties are involved (combined therapy), the cost to the patient can be discouraging. Seldom, if ever, is any of it covered by dental insurance. The majority of cases, however, do not involve all of these specialties, and the cost is quite manageable if you look at it as an investment in health, comfort, self-esteem, and the enjoyment of old age.

You may well ask "What is the best way to deal with the cost problem?" Since there is no form of insurance available to cover these costs, it also seems unlikely that shrinking medicare services will be expanded to include it, so what should you do? See DENTAL INSURANCE (Chapter 14).

The answer to that question is entirely personal and depends largely on what has already been done to save the teeth. For those people who place a high value on their teeth, which is likely to include you, the answer is to plan for it. The need for oral reconstruction should not be a surprise, nor viewed as a curse or individual weakness. The thought of losing their teeth is a serious psychological trauma for many people. Decisions regarding this procedure should be made only with the aid of a competent dentist and based on a thorough dental diagnosis. If in doubt, don't hesitate to get an entirely independent second opinion, just as you would for any major elective surgery. Cost should be viewed with regard to long-term benefits (amortized over the remaining lifetime) and competence should not be confused with salesmanship. ✜

Chapter 11

COSMETIC DENTISTRY

Your smile is one of your most important assets. Most people know this instinctively. Henry Miller, a highly respected writer of this century, has this to say about smiles. "When you speak to people—smile. It is a wonderful thing when you meet someone and they just instinctively smile and say 'I am mighty glad to know you.' There is power in a smile. It is one of the best relaxation exercises of which I know."

Since your teeth are the most visible evidence of your smile, it is important to have them appear as nearly perfect as possible. With bonded veneers, new tooth-whitening techniques, and simplified orthodontics, your dentist can make remarkable improvements in your smile. Depending on the severity of the problem, the treatment can be simple, involving adhesive fillings, tooth-whitening, or bonded veneers. Or, it may be more complex, requiring orthodontia and in some cases, major jaw surgery.

A good example of the radical changes possible may be remembered by those who watched Carol Burnett on TV over the years. Despite the need for orthodontia, she rose to the top of her field as an entertainer; more credit to her! But, like most of us who want to enjoy the power of our smile, she decided to do something. The result was a remarkable improvement in her smile.

Since your smile is so important to your self-image, it is not surprising that the major concern of most patients is cosmetic dentistry. As just mentioned, there are many new techniques and improved materials for achieving aesthetic results never before possible.

Tooth-whitening agents and techniques are now available that are more effective than older, less-reliable methods usually referred to as bleaching. Some depend on mild abrasives to remove surface stains; others use chemicals to change the color of the enamel and underlying dentin. Your dentist will know which one is best for your particular problem.

Adhesive, light-cured composite resins are used for fillings and reshaping teeth to a natural attractive appearance. Because this approach requires little or no cutting of the teeth, it is painless, and the results are often dramatic. But, their durability and resistance to stains are not as good as baked porcelain.

Bonded veneers made of baked porcelain are used to cover unsightly teeth and restore them to a normal and attractive appearance with the color of your choice; these days you may have your teeth as white as you wish (Fig. 12).

Porcelain crowns are not new; for years they

BAKED PORCELAIN VENEER FOR FRACTURED INCISOR

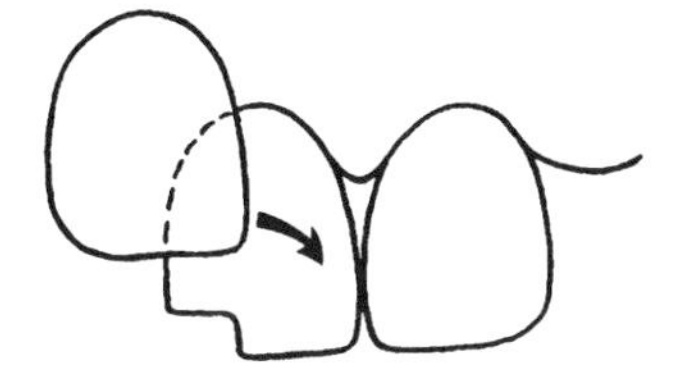

Figure 12

have been the keystone of cosmetic dentistry. But, there are improved methods of fabrication that make them more resistant to fracture and more natural in appearance.

Orthodontic therapy, the basic procedure for straightening crooked teeth, has been streamlined with new materials that enable dentists to make braces almost invisible. If the braces can do their job worn on the inside tooth surfaces, they are completely invisible! Modern brace design has enabled dentists to cut orthodontic treatment time in half, and today there are nearly as many adult patients, of all ages, having their teeth straightened as there are children.

Orthognathic surgery makes it possible to correct facial deformities and repair serious injuries to the face as the result of accidents. Dentists who do this are maxillofacial surgeons, highly trained specialists who combine the skills required of dental, orthopedic, and cosmetic surgeons.

Oral reconstruction is the ultimate answer for restoring aesthetics to a badly broken down dentition; in mouths where many teeth are missing, weakened by decay or worn-out fillings, discolored or disfigured by systemic disease, or simply worn out and discolored due to age (a common problem as our longevity increases). This procedure usually requires rebuilding all the teeth in a coordinated treatment plan with the goal of restoring the dentition to a highly cosmetic appearance along with normal dental function. It provides some of the best examples of dental artistry and makes one aware of the many skills that must be mastered by dentists who provide these complex services.

A word of caution about dental aesthetics. There is no doubt about the truth of the old saw—beauty is in the eye of the beholder. Many people think that the whiter the teeth, the prettier the smile. In a young person this is generally true. But time ages teeth as it does everything else. Years of drinking tea, coffee, red wine, colored fruit juices, salad dressings, and lots of deliciously seasoned foods cause teeth to darken very gradually, to show lines of stress or mini-fractures in the enamel, and to appear worn. In the same time period, hair changes to gray and then to white, skin becomes wrinkled and mottled, and facial tissues change. To restore teeth to the white, unworn appearance that they had in youth often makes them stand out as artifacts in a mature face. It is usually much more appropriate to only lighten teeth rather than whiten them, and to reduce the worn appearance rather than eliminate it completely when reconstructing the dentition of a person over the age of 50 or 60, depending on the amount of discoloration and wear present in the natural teeth. But, with due respect for the eye of the beholder, the final choice must be left to the patient, who, it must be remembered, is the one to be pleased. ✤

Chapter 12

HOW TO CHOOSE YOUR DENTIST

Advertising pays! How else would you explain the billions of dollars spent every year for advertising in newspapers, radio, TV, billboards, yellow pages, newsletters, catalogs, junk mail, etc.? Every student of business administration is taught the importance of public relations and the effectiveness of innovative advertising techniques in a competitive world. And much of the advertising is based on the statement made by P. T. Barnum many years ago: "There's a sucker born every minute." Of course, not all advertising should be painted with this broad tar brush, but there is a lot of evidence to prove that much of it strains the limits of truthfulness. Sorting out the truth, the misleading statements, and the outright lies is the challenge every buyer of goods and services faces daily.

The range of these choices is extreme; from homes and automobiles at the high end to the simple purchase of a package of aspirin tablets (often needed to relieve the headache generated by the other purchases). Medical and dental services are somewhere in the middle; choosing a dentist will be more difficult for a person who places a high value on his or her dental health and appearance than for one whose priorities do not include dental health. For those who care about their well-being, common sense tells them to be selective in choosing their dentists.

There is a popular misconception that because a person has a degree from an accredited school of dentistry (yes, there are some foreign schools that are not accredited in the U.S.), he or she is well qualified to provide dental services. Signing to their names D.D.S. (Doctor of Dental Surgery), or D.M.D. (Doctor of Medicine in Dentistry), depending on the school from which they graduated, means only that they have completed a basic training course in the fundamentals of dental knowledge and practice. The time required to gain that degree varies from six to eight years, depending on the requirements of the school and the abilities of the student.

Before they may work for the public and charge a fee for their services, the graduates must pass a state licensing examination that usually takes three days. This leads to another misconception; because this person has been licensed by the state, he or she must be well qualified.

It is true that strict educational requirements and licensing are important measures intended to protect the public from abusive treatment, serious bodily harm, and exploitation by charlatans. But this is the same standard of protection offered by the state for many other services, medical and non-medical, all of which require a license to do business. It is also true that physicians and dentists are supposed to adhere to a higher code of ethics and are held responsible by their professional organizations to maintain high standards of practice. But that tradition has been weakened by the fact that today it is legal and considered not unethical for a dentist to advertise. And no licensed dentist may be denied admission to his or her local dental society without due cause.

How safe are these elaborate testing and licensing requirements, this "safety net," to use the expression of politicians who administer it? From the amount of litigation and number of complaints about malpractice, it would seem to be not very effective. We hear all about the disappointments, bad results, or calamities that may result from dental treatment because the media are quick to present negative news and seldom give the positive side of this picture equal time. Millions of dental procedures are completed every day with the total satisfaction of patient and dentist! In a public-opinion poll rating professional and business services for integrity, dentists were at the top of the list; above physicians and all other professions. (Lawyers, to no one's surprise, were far down the list.)

Despite this presumption of safety and protection from abuse, it is wise to choose your dentist carefully; the more you value your teeth and smile the more choosy you should be. You should not pick your dentist from the yellow pages. If you "Let your fingers do the walking" to pick your dentist, your teeth may walk away with them. What people advertise may not be what they deliver. Words can be misleading; implied guarantees in the field of medicine are considered unethical because the human body is so complex and biological responses are so variable. Advertising as a tool for recruiting new patients has always been taboo in medicine and it should remain so. The best advertising for a doctor is word of mouth. Firsthand reports of satisfied patients are your best leads in choosing your dentist. Firsthand reports of dissatisfied patients are usually equally valid. Notice the emphasis on "firsthand reports." Hearsay is subject to exaggeration and misinterpretation and may not be very reliable.

The routine suggestion given for selecting a doctor is to call the local medical or dental society (a branch of the American Dental Association) for a recommendation. This can be helpful. Usually you will receive the names of two or three dentists who are respected members. But because the law now says membership must be open to all licensed dentists, you are not getting the benefit of personal evaluation that comes from speaking to the doctors' patients. Moreover, the people you would ask, presumably your friends and acquaintances, are likely to share your values and opinions. The dentist who pleases them is likely to meet with your approval too.

When it comes to selecting a dental specialist (surgeon, orthodontist, periodontist, etc.), you should rely on your family (general) dentist. Specialists in your area should be recommended by someone who respects and works with them every day; one who knows their qualifications and status as "board certified."

One additional source of information about the qualifications of the general dentist you are seeking may be the roster of members of the Academy of General Dentistry (AGD). This national organization is dedicated to promoting advanced, postgraduate training for general dentists. There are many short courses sponsored by dental schools and other interested groups to help dentists update their knowledge and improve their skills in every field of practice. Members of the AGD report the courses they have taken and when they have accumulated the required number of credits in the various fields of dentistry, with accredited teachers, they are honored at a yearly convocation and become Fellows of the Academy of General Dentistry. They may then add "FAGD" to the DDS in their signature and sign DDS, FAGD.

These two degrees signify that they have completed requirements for recognition of advanced education. At an even higher level of training, with many more units of postgraduate education required, a "Fellow" may advance to "Master" and then sign MAGD instead of FAGD. The odds are good that a general dentist who has achieved the recognition of the AGD (FAGD or MAGD) is likely to provide high standards of dental service.

In any case, if the dentist you choose does not establish a feeling of concern for your dental health, along with good rapport so that you consider him or her your friend, it is probably wise to seek another dentist. Don't allow yourself to become a faceless number in a dental production line—a cog in a money machine. ✜

Chapter 13

PREVENTION

Sir Walter Raleigh is remembered for having thrown his cloak on the mud so that the queen could walk over the puddle and not mess up her shoes; the epitome of a gentleman. He is less well-remembered, if at all, for his idea of prevention. In a letter written to his friend Robert Cecil, dated May 10, 1593, he wrote, "Prevention is the daughter of intelligence." Certainly, the relationship is clear. By extension, good health is the daughter of prevention and the granddaughter of intelligence.

When we think of prevention, we mean to avoid the problem entirely or at least stop it before it gets serious, the earlier the better. In the case of teeth, early is the 42nd day of pregnancy, when the tooth buds begin to develop. So here is just another example of why pregnant women should be careful about their diet, along with avoiding smoking, alcohol, and drugs. Fluoride, in the proper quantity (ask your dentist), can help develop decay-resistant teeth. After childbirth, fluorides added to the infant's diet, again in proper quantities depending on your drinking water analysis, help build strong teeth. In the absence of any visible dental problems, nothing else needs to be added to your child's diet to promote healthy teeth.

Brushing and flossing are irrelevant in this early stage of tooth development, but children like to imitate their parents, even at that early age, so if brushing seems like fun, it is not too early to establish the habit, however uncoordinated it may be.

Somewhere between the ages of three and five it is wise to introduce your child to the family dentist or to a pedodontist, a dentist who specializes in children's dentistry. Early diagnosis and treatment of existing or impending problems is the primary goal of your dentist, and with his or her help, you will see your child grow up with perfect teeth and a beautiful smile. As a mature adult, it will then be his or her responsibility to maintain it. This gets us back to the quote at the beginning of this chapter, "Prevention is the daughter of intelligence" and, by extension, good health is the daughter of prevention.

If this emphasis on intelligence seems logical, as it is, consider the reasoning of someone who smokes cigarettes or consumes large quantities of alcoholic beverages or takes drugs intravenously or is sexually promiscuous or is grossly overweight or lives on junk foods, oblivious of dietary needs and the consequences of ignoring them. Participants in all these unhealthy practices try to explain their actions with what they consider good reasons; but none of the reasons passes the test of intelligence.

The fact is that we tend to take good health for granted. We shun medical and dental treatment; it invades our privacy, and it is human to follow the easiest path through life with the attitude, "If it ain't broke, don't fix it." We wait for symptoms before we consult a doctor. Or, we buy billions of dollars' worth of over-the-counter remedies to avoid consulting a doctor. Many people wait until a disease is serious or life-threatening before they begin to consider prevention in an effort to avoid a relapse or recurrence. Look at the men jogging after a coronary bypass who were too busy to do so before the surgery. Most heavy smokers unable to quit smoking before they are diagnosed with lung cancer become able to do so afterward.

Medical science has unraveled many of the threads that combine to make up the complicated biological mechanism we call a human being. We have learned much about the care and maintenance of this complex machine. Applying that knowledge is a challenge to the intelligence of each individual, and it imposes a burden of self-discipline. Accepting that challenge and assuming that burden is the key to prevention of disease and the enjoyment of good health.

The good news is that almost all dental diseases are preventable. By using intelligence and self-discipline in applying a few simple rules, you can protect yourself from dental disease and the loss of your teeth. Here they are, listed in order of importance:

Rule 1. Learn to be meticulous about your oral hygiene. This involves more than waving a toothbrush at your teeth on a haphazard schedule. My assistant, who teaches oral hygiene to our patients, has considered making a video tape to enter in "The Funniest Home Movies" contest. The antics of people when asked to show how they brush their teeth are often regrettably laughable. Oral hygiene is much more than toothbrushing. Rather than toothbrushing, think of oral hygiene as "mouthcleaning" or "gumbrushing." A proper procedure is explained in ORAL HYGIENE IS NUMBER ONE (Chapter 3). To be sure you are doing it correctly, check with your dentist or dental hygienist. They will also advise you on the use of fluorides in the form of toothpaste, mouthwash, or special gels. Fluorides for the prevention of tooth decay have been proven effective and should be used regularly, but because there is a slight danger of fluoride poisoning if large quantities are consumed, dentists are required to prescribe products that contain more than the very small quantities found in almost all toothpastes and over-the-counter oral hygiene products.

Rule 2. Have regular dental checkups at least once a year. This is a good time to review your oral hygiene procedures by demonstration. We all tend to backslide in this routine. Many patients require periodic retraining to stay on track with their oral hygiene. An x-ray examination should be made to look for new cavities at least every two years at checkup appointments. A full-mouth x-ray examination every five years is usually recommended. These intervals may be changed by your dentist if you have special problems that need more frequent checkups.

Rule 3. Adjust your diet to the needs of your body, not to the whims of flavor, fad, or convenience. Your genes and daily activities dictate the quantity of food you need, the types of food you tolerate well, and the way they are processed in your body. The hackneyed advice of "Eat a well-balanced diet" says nothing about total quantities, method of preparation, or best sources of the foods you consume. Milk is an excellent source of dietary calcium, but feeding children lots of milk is no guarantee they will have perfect teeth. How do you choose among non-fat, 2% fat, regular (4%) fat, chocolate milk, and buttermilk? Many people can drink any or all of these milk products in moderation with no ill effects; others cannot tolerate any of them and may need goat's milk as a source of calcium. Similar decisions must be made in selecting all types of food, and new products keep coming into the market competing for your food dollars.

The standard bugaboo, excessive consumption of refined carbohydrates (candy, ice cream, soft drinks, sugared breakfast foods, cookies, cake, and pie), seems to be little or no deterrent to the manufacture of these products, which means there must be a market for them. However, they also offer all of these goodies sweetened with artificial sweeteners and advertise them as sugar-free. The controversy over the long term effects of artificial sweeteners adds confusion to a problem that is already complicated for many health-conscious parents. There is a certain amount of overkill in this area which leads to unnecessary feelings of guilt or frustration. Small quantities of sugar used in cooking as a seasoning may add to the taste of food without any danger of causing tooth decay.

It is important to learn to read labels on packaged foods. Because the contents are listed in their order of percentage of the total ingredients, when sugar is mentioned first or second on the list of contents, you know that the product has a high content of sugar. The presence of sugar is not a reason for avoiding any food, if it is consumed as part of a regular meal. It is the eating of snacks between meals, many of which are highly sugared, that contributes in a major way to tooth decay.

For ongoing guidance about diet and nutrition I suggest a subscription to one of the many reputable newsletters published by schools of nutrition at leading universities. See Appendix B.

Rule 4. Using your teeth to crack nuts, open bottles, and chew ice puts you at risk of fracturing tooth enamel. Expensive dental procedures may be needed to save the broken tooth—or teeth. Chewing gum is a bad habit. It accelerates the wearing out of teeth and the TMJ may become overstressed and painful.

Rule 5. Crooked teeth are difficult to keep clean and usually do not provide good chewing function. They should be straightened; orthodontia usually can be done at any age. If in doubt, ask your family dentist to refer you to an orthodontist. Many young children (6 to 12) may avoid major orthodontia by early preventive treatment, called interceptive orthodontia.

Rule 6. Missing teeth should be replaced with a fixed prosthesis (bridgework) whenever possible in order to prevent the collapse of the dental arch and the loss of more teeth. Alternative procedures may be recommended by your dentist depending on the individual problem. After careful consideration, the necessary restorations should be completed.

Rule 7. If you smoke or chew tobacco, kick these habits. Cancer of the mouth is a high price to pay for this offensive (to most non-smokers) behavior. And, as mentioned in MOUTH INFECTIONS (Chapter 7), the use of drugs and promiscuous sex can lead to serious diseases such as AIDS, which may make their first appearance in the mouth.

Rule 8. If you clench your jaws or grind your teeth, usually while sleeping (check with your sleeping partner), consult your dentist for help in overcoming this habit (bruxism). It can destroy your teeth's chewing surfaces, cause fractures, and accelerate the need for major oral reconstruction and its attendant expenses.

Common sense dictates other rules which you should follow as the needs arise. In any case, you must make the rules fit into your lifestyle or adjust your lifestyle to fit the rules. The goal is prevention of dental disease and the enjoyment of teeth for your lifetime. ✣

Chapter 14

COSTS VERSUS BENEFITS

The president of a local manufacturing company, highly respected for his business success, was consulting me about new dentures. Looking at him for the first time, I was shocked by the appearance of his facial profile and his teeth. His face looked as if his chin was trying to meet his nose; the way old people look when they have no teeth. In the cartoon world he would be Popeye. When he smiled, his teeth jumped out at you, pearly white and in a nice straight row, like a picket fence. It was obvious to me that he was wearing worn-out, ill-fitting dentures. But he did not think so. The only reason he came in was because they were cracked, for the fourth time, and he was beginning to think they should be replaced. When I asked him if they were loose or painful, he replied, "Yes, but I've been wearing them twenty years and have gotten used to them." After we talked about what caused him to get full dentures at the age of forty and the amount of pain and discomfort he has suffered since, he came up with

George Burns' one liner, "If I had known I was going to live so long, I'd have taken better care of myself."

The reason he gave for opting for full dentures was the cost of fixing his natural teeth. He was just getting established in his business and felt the treatment plan his denist had proposed was beyond his budget and too expensive. When I told him about the cost of new dentures, and the fact that they too would eventually need to be replaced, with the need to accommodate and adjust to them each time, he asked about dental implants. Yes, he was a good candidate for dental implants, but when that extra cost was explained to him, he remarked that to get them now would more than wipe out any savings afforded by dentures. And the pain and discomfort he had suffered over the years were no bonus. He finally came to the sad realization that no amount of money saved could buy new natural teeth.

The recent advances in dental implants come close to doing that, but they are suitable only if you have the right amount and type of bone structure and the pocketbook to pay the cost. When considering costs, we must add the investment of time and effort required to keep them clean and free of infection. Implants are more susceptible to infection than natural teeth because they have no biological tissue seal (as natural teeth do) against the army of bacteria that parades through the mouth. Keeping implants clean requires even more meticulous everyday care than with natural teeth.

This leads to some interesting statistics about the "high" cost of dentistry. Let's begin by describing the "ideal" patient. Mr. and Mrs.

Cleanteeth are twenty years old, at the age when they begin to take full responsibility for their own health; they have had several fillings in their back teeth, as most teenagers do; they have had their teeth straightened; they do not chew gum, smoke or chew tobacco, or drink sweetened soft drinks; they brush their gums, teeth, and tongue, and floss between their teeth every day after breakfast and before bedtime; they have had their wisdom teeth removed; they have not lost any other teeth due to accidents or dental neglect; they have attractive smiles and want to keep them that way—for their lifetime! Being sensible young people, they listen to the conventional wisdom and get a dental checkup at least once a year. They have their teeth cleaned, including cavity-revealing x-rays, once a year and have full-mouth x-rays every five years. If there is a need for repairs due to decay or gum disease, they take care of it promptly, and they follow their dentist's suggestions in order to avoid a recurrence. If a tooth is lost as the result of an accident, they have it replaced. This is preventive dentistry—the best way to make sure that your teeth last for your lifetime. It is also the least costly.

At present-day dental fees, a recall appointment for tooth cleaning, hygiene instruction, and x-ray checkup costs $75 to $100. While the services may be provided by a dental hygienist, the dentist should confer with the hygienist and make sure nothing is overlooked. It takes a minimum of thirty minutes and more often forty-five minutes or an hour to complete a thorough dental checkup. Dental offices and clinics that advertise cut rates for this important procedure are not likely to spend enough time or give proper emphasis to prevention; they are more interested in the larger fees associated with other treatments.

Over a period of forty years, our model patients are now sixty and grandparents. For each, the total expenditure for dental care may be as low as $4,000 ($100 per year per person), not adjusted for inflation. This is an achievable goal that has been verified by examining the records of several hundred patients in one private-practice office. But, this result is not the rule, nor even average.

Most people do not have the benefit of the good beginnings that we gave Mr. and Mrs. Cleanteeth, and we are all victims of accidents that often involve injury to the teeth. But neglect and lack of motivation are the most common causes of major dental expense. In the absence of serious symptoms of dental disease, such as toothache, bleeding gums, or extraction for infected teeth, most people enjoy the comfort of "if it ain't broke, don't fix it." They prefer to avoid the inconvenience of "if you want it to last longer, take good care of it."

Compare the cost of maintaining a reasonably healthy mouth from youth to old age at $100 per year to the cost of rebuilding or restoring one tooth at a cost of $500. ($500 per tooth is the average fee in today's dental market). If you had to have all twenty-eight teeth restored with full crowns, it would total $14,000. Many people spend that much over a period of forty years just in emergency or patch-up repairs. In either case, you are likely to arrive at the age of 60 or 70 with teeth that are in need of rebuilding if they are to last another twenty years, which is not uncommon, given our extended life spans. Where do you get the $14,000 needed to rebuild them? You can be sure medicare won't pay the bill. And there is no insurance program now available to help you meet that expense.

It has been my experience that there are only two types of patients able to cope with this problem comfortably. One is the relatively small group who have accumulated or inherited wealth and who don't flinch at any expense if it will add to their comfort and enjoyment of life. They are sometimes referred to as "the rich and famous." For them, the dental expense is a minor consideration. They are usually most interested in appearance and may pay $20,000 to $30,000 for this service. The other group is made up of people who, after a lifetime of productive work and saving for retirement, find themselves with a nice financial cushion that more than meets their needs. They have planned well enough to absorb the shock of this major expense and use their money to provide comfort and pleasure in their old age. Many people, however, say they cannot afford it.

The benefits of natural teeth cannot be measured in dollars. The rich and famous of the world would all have natural teeth if they could be purchased for money. In the early part of this century, dentistry was still in the dark ages of extraction and dentures. For some people, that still seems to be the case. But with today's sophisticated dental technology it does not have to happen to you. Practice prevention and plan for reconstruction. You should not expect that this major expense will ever be covered by any dental insurance plan.

Dental insurance is considered by many people a big bonanza provided by benevolent employers or a caretaker government. It has been very useful in encouraging people to take care of their teeth and improve their general health. Before there was dental insurance most working people went to the dentist only when they had a toothache or some obvious dental problem. Regular dental care was an "expensive" luxury, not a necessity. Serious dental problems were solved by extracting all the teeth and replacing them with dentures, no matter what the age of the patient.

I cannot forget the high-school principal who brought his sixteen-year-old daughter with rampant tooth caries (decay in almost all her teeth) to my office and asked me to extract all her teeth and to replace them with full dentures. After recovering from shock, I suggested filling the cavities, changing her diet, and instructing her in dental hygiene as the proper way to treat this unfortunate child. Of course, the cost was not insignificant. But it would cost just as much for the extractions and dentures. When I refused to go along with his insistence on the dentures route (in his myopic view, to eliminate future expense), he chose to seek another dentist who would cooperate with his wishes. I do not know the final outcome.

Cruel as it seems today, this attitude was not uncommon just forty years ago. In some areas it still persists. The fact that the reverse is generally true and that most people can now look forward to retaining at least some of their teeth for their lifetime is due to the advances in dental science (fluorides, antibiotics, improved materials and techniques) and the wider use of dental services encouraged by dental insurance programs.

Dental insurance has been a big plus for public health. Thanks to dental insurance, many people who would otherwise neglect their teeth until they experienced pain are now seeing their dentists at regular intervals. They are practicing prevention. They are more aware of the importance of daily oral hygiene and the role of nutrition in dental health. Health consciousness, in general, has been raised, and with the financial burden seemingly eased by insurance, patients have been able to retain teeth that might otherwise have been extracted.

I say "seemingly eased by insurance" because the negative side of dental insurance is difficult to present and most people don't want to hear it. The notion that dental insurance provides high-quality services at less cost is misleading. The highest level of dental care can be provided only with a doctor-patient relationship in which the doctor accepts responsibility for the quality of his or her services (not to be taken for granted, as it often is) and the patient accepts responsibility for the fees, regardless of third-party reimbursement plans (insurance). Like every other group of providers, dentists vary in competence and integrity. Competent dentists take pride in having helped their patients retain their teeth for their lifetime. No dental insurance plan can do it without them. Costs and benefits of dental care are definitely related and widely misunderstood. ✥

Chapter 15

DENTISTRY IN THE FUTURE

Science is advancing at such a rapid pace on all fronts that any predictions of things to come are likely to be understatements. Space-age technology spreads to every field of human activity; industry, home, work, and recreation as fast as it is discovered. Dental scientists are quick to apply the new knowledge to solve dental problems and improve dental health. And the media are just as prompt in reporting whatever seems like "hot news." That's their job. But TV personalities, talk-show hosts, and Hollywood celebrities are not scientists, and their efforts to report scientific facts are often distorted by their desire to raise their ratings. A story aired by CBS on "60 Minutes" exemplifies this careless attitude. It is important to be aware that this is likely to continue in the future as long as it is profitable.

The condemnation of silver amalgam as a dental filling material because it contains mercury has never been justified based on extensive scientific research by dental scientists in dental schools and research institutes worldwide. These investigations have been ongoing for many years without any corroborating evidence of mercury poisoning. Amalgam fillings have been placed in the mouths of millions of patients with no indication of mercury poisoning. The mercury in dental amalgam is combined with silver and zinc in a form that makes it insoluble in water or saliva. It has been said by experienced metallurgists that if the mercury leaked out of the amalgam as suggested by the notoriety seekers, the fillings would wash out of the teeth over a period of time less than ten years, no matter how slowly it deteriorated. Yet we see routinely in dentistry amalgam fillings that have been in the mouths of healthy patients for over thirty years. That fact alone is reason enough to dismiss any efforts to condemn its usefulness as a dental filling material. True, it has disadvantages compared to gold or tooth-colored filling materials but its low cost relative to other materials has made it the traditional choice of cost-conscious patients.

There is no doubt that mercury itself is a dangerous poison. The people at most risk for this are those engaged in purifying it for industrial purposes and who use it in manufacturing processes. In dental offices the people at risk are the dental assistant and the dentist, who may be exposed to these vapors repeatedly over a long period of time if they handle the mercury carelessly when combining it with silver alloy for placement in the mouth. Dentists know this full well, and you may be sure careful dentists see to it that no free mercury accumulates in their offices to vaporize and affect their own health or that of their staffs.

Getting back to the progress of science and its effect on the future of dentistry, we may classify it in two broad areas; biochemical and mechanical. Biochemistry, which gave dentistry fluorides, will some day provide vaccines for control and prevention of dental decay and periodontal disease. This work, which has been going on for many years, will make increasing progress as we better understand gene-splicing and auto-immune disease. Biochemistry also gave us composite resins and ceramic products that can be bonded to enamel and dentin and which have caused a revolution in restorative dentistry; the business of filling teeth and making them look good with minimum discomfort to the patient. Here are some prospects for major advances that I see happening in the next decade.

Anti-plaque chemicals, which we have now, will be improved and will help ensure that periodontal disease, the number one threat to teeth, becomes entirely controllable.

Vaccines targeted to the specific bacteria that cause dental decay will help prevent and control this number two dental disease. A chemical in green tea has been found to destroy streptococcus mutans, the bacterium that plays a major role in dental decay. You can look forward to being bombarded with green-tea toothpaste, chewing gum, and mouthwash along with the traditional Chinese restaurant dessert, green-tea ice cream.

Farther into the future, gene-splicing and monoclonal antibody research which holds out hope for control of cancer, herpes, and many diseases resistant to treatment, will include all the diseases that appear in the mouth.

Transplantation of embryonic tooth tissues

(tooth buds), a technique that has had very limited success to date, will become a viable form of replacement for missing teeth. This idea, which is not original with me, goes back to the time when I was a senior student in dental school (1936) and did a research study which was published with the impressive title "Heterotopic Transplantation of Permanent Tooth Germ in the Cat." It didn't work, but we know a lot more about it today than we did then.

Implantation of fabricated parts (implants) into the bone of the jaws to simulate or replace teeth, a technique now in its infancy, will become routine as sophisticated new materials and biological techniques are perfected.

On the mechanical side, we now have a machine that removes decayed tooth material, records the shape of the resultant preparation in the tooth, and fabricates gold fillings and crowns; a robot that makes precision-fit dental restorations. This computer-aided design and computer-aided manufacture (CAD-CAM) system combines modern sensing techniques, computer enhancement, and electronically controlled milling equipment.

A jaw movement simulator is a machine that senses and reproduces the complex movement of the lower jaw as it is related to the upper jaw. This information is important in the process of oral reconstruction because each individual has a pattern of jaw movement just as unique as fingerprints. For the past thirty years the dentists who use this information (gnathologists) have relied on an analog computer to create these records. More recently, they have developed electronic devices that work with a digital computer to obtain this important data. As the technique is improved with the aid of electronics, computers, and bioengineering, it will be used more widely to meet the very precise requirements of oral reconstruction.

The use of lasers in medicine is becoming routine, even though it has been just a few years since this technology was in its infancy and referred to most often when discussing "star wars." Today it is used in dental surgery mostly by periodontists and, as the equipment is improved and costs decrease, lasers will become routine dental office equipment.

Bonding has revolutionized aesthetics in dentistry. The ability to fill cavities, restore broken teeth, and cover eroded areas with tooth-colored composite resins has made dentistry much more acceptable to many people.

This technology, a product of spacecraft design, is being constantly upgraded, and every improvement is quickly adapted to dental needs. The competition between baked porcelain and composite resins is ongoing and challenging. Each has advantages and disadvantages for dental restorative purposes, and choosing among them is a matter that should be discussed with your dentist. The decision will depend on the type of restoration being considered and the latest improvements in these materials.

Baked porcelain has been the material of choice for maximum aesthetic effect for many years, but its fragility and brittleness make it unsuitable for stress-bearing restorations, especially on chewing surfaces. Cast porcelain is new. It is stronger and less brittle, and as it is improved it may gain wider acceptance. Composite resins are also being improved to make them more wear-resistant and unaffected by saliva. Their ease of handling gives them a large advantage over porcelain; usually they are applied directly to the teeth and cured (hardened) with a high-intensity light transmitted by fiber optics.

Summarizing the future of dentistry, it is likely that the biological sciences will make prevention of dental disease routine. At the same time, the extension of our life span will make ever more important the process of oral reconstruction, which will become necessary for most of us who live to seventy and beyond. To meet this need, the fabrication of replacement teeth and the materials for making them will be constantly up-graded, and what is now reasonably acceptable will be replaced by a higher standard of aesthetics and durability. The human dentition, which plays a key role in nutrition, health, beauty, and self-esteem, and which is unique in the body's inability to maintain or restore it by normal healing processes, will be kept in normal function for the ever-increasing life span of future generations by the advances in dental science in the hands of skillful dentists. There is a bright future for those dental scientists, dentists, and patients who are committed to the concept of teeth for a lifetime. ✤

Appendix A

DENTAL HYGIENE AIDS

Oral hygiene aids are useful when they are recognized as "aids" and not as substitutes for motivation or attention to detail. The best route to a clean mouth is patient motivation. The wide array of toothbrushes, toothpastes, and dental floss offered to the public to "improve" oral hygiene is bewildering simply because every commercial opportunity is used to accommodate some real or imagined special need for maintaining dental health.

The basic tools for oral hygiene have long been recognized as the toothbrush, toothpaste, and dental floss. In the light of current knowledge about plaque control, add to these a wooden toothpick mounted in a handle that makes it possible to reach every area of the teeth, front and back. Some periodontists rate the toothpick first, above all the other oral-hygiene aids.

Because oral hygiene is big business and manufacturers tend to get carried away with claims for their effectiveness, the American Dental Association conducts an ongoing program of monitoring, testing, and evaluating oral-hygiene products and devices in order to help the dental profession make recommendations based on scientific research and to protect the consumer from false or unsupported claims.

The products listed below have been evaluated by the ADA's Council on Dental Therapeutics and Council on Dental Materials, Instruments and Equipment, and have earned the Seal of Acceptance of the American Dental Association.

MANUAL TOOTHBRUSHES

Aim Toothbrush, Cheseborough-Pond's Inc.
Arco Toothbrush, Arco International
Butler Toothbrushes, John O. Butler Co.
Colgate Jr. Toothbrush, Colgate-Palmolive Co.
Colgate Toothbrushes, Colgate-Palmolive Co.
Dental H Toothbrush, Dental Hygiene Co.
Dentax Toothbrush, Carewell Industries
Disney Toothbrushes, Lever Research & Development
Hugger Toothbrush, Hugger Corporation
Improve Toothbrush, Prevent Care Products, Inc.
Lactona Toothbrushes, Lactona Corp.
McDonald Toothbrush, Performance Concepts
Milor Angle Plus Toothbrush, Milor Corp.
Milor Angle Toothbrush, Milor Corp.
Milor Toothbrush, Milor Corp.
Oral-B Toothbrushes, Oral-B Laboratories
Oral-B Ultra, Oral-B Laboratories
Pepsodent Plus Toothbrush, Cheseborough-Pond's Inc.
Pepsodent Toothbrushes, Cheseborough-Pond's Inc.
Prevent Toothbrush, Johnson & Johnson Professional Care Co.

Py-Co-Pay Softex Toothbrushes, Block Drug Co., Inc.
Py-Co-Twin Brush, Block Drug Co., Inc.
Reach Gentle Toothbrush, Johnson & Johnson Professional Care Co.
Reach Toothbrushes, Johnson & Johnson Professional Care Co.
Sensodyne Gentle Toothbrushes, Block Drug Co., Inc.
Sensodyne Search Toothbrushes, Block Drug Co., Inc.

FLUORIDE DENTIFRICES

Aqua-fresh Tartar Control Toothpaste, Beecham Products
Check-Up Plaque-Removing Fluoride Tooth Gel, Rydelle-Lion, Inc.
Check-Up Plaque-Removing Fluoride Toothpaste, Rydelle-Lion, Inc.
Colgate Fluoride Gel, Colgate-Palmolive Co.
Colgate Fluoride Toothpaste, Colgate-Palmolive Co.
Colgate Tartar Control Formula Gel, Colgate-Palmolive Co.
Colgate Tartar Control Formula Toothpaste, Colgate-Palmolive Co.
Crest Double Action Toothpaste, Proctor & Gamble Co.
Crest Tartar Control Formula Toothpaste, Mint, Regular, Proctor & Gamble Co.
Crest Toothpaste, Mint, Regular, Proctor & Gamble Co.
Crest Toothpaste for Kids, Super Cool Gel, Proctor & Gamble Co.
Gel Formula Crest, Proctor & Gamble Co.

Muppets Fluoride Toothpaste, Bubble Gum, Mild Mint, Oral-B Laboratories
Sesame Street Fluoride Toothpaste, Oral-B Laboratories
Anti-Tartar Aim Plus Fluoride Toothpaste, Cheseborough-Pond's Inc.
Aqua-Fresh Fluoride Toothpaste, Cheseborough-Pond's Inc.
Aqua Fresh for Kids, Beecham Products
Colgate Junior with MFP Fluoride Gel, Colgate-Palmolive Co.
Colgate with MFP Fluoride Gel, Colgate-Palmolive Co.
Colgate with MFP Fluoride Toothpaste, Colgate-Palmolive Co.
Dentagard Fluoride Toothpaste, Colgate-Palmolive Co.
Extra-Strength Aim Gel, Cheseborough-Pond's Inc.
Extra Strength Aim Toothpaste, Cheseborough-Pond's Inc.
Macleans Fluoride Toothpaste, Mildmint, Peppermint, Beecham Products
Regular-Strength Aim Toothpaste, Mint, Regular, Cheseborough-Pond's Inc.
Zact H-P Toothpaste, Rydelle-Lion Inc.
Zact Smoker's Gel, Rydelle-Lion Inc.
Zact Smoker's Toothpaste, Rydelle-Lion Inc.

DESENSITIZING DENTIFRICES

Denquel Sensitive Teeth Toothpaste, Proctor & Gamble Co.
Mint Sensodyne Toothpaste for Sensitive Teeth, Block Drug Co. Inc.
Promise Toothpaste for Sensitive Teeth, Block Drug Co., Inc.
Protect Toothpaste for Sensitive Teeth, John O. Butler Co.

Sensodyne Toothpaste for Sensitive Teeth, Block Drug Co., Inc.

FLUORIDE MOUTHWASHES
(over the counter)

ACT Anti-Cavity Dental Rinse, Johnson & Johnson Prof. Dental Care Co.
Fluorigard Anti-Cavity Dental Rinse, Colgate-Palmolive Co.
Ghostbusters Anti-Cavity Dental Rinse, Perio Products
Kolynos Fluoride Dental Rinse, Whitehall-Boyle International
Reach Fluoride Dental Rinse, Johnson & Johnson Professional Dental Care Co.

ORAL IRRIGATING DEVICES

Dento-Spray, Texell Products
Gum Machine, Gum Machine Co.
Propulse 7618, Propulse Inc.
Sunbeam Models 6271, 6272 (Provisionally Acceptable), Northern Electric
Co.Water Pik, Teledyne Water Pik

POWERED ORAL-HYGIENE DEVICES

Braun Appliances, Braun, Inc.
Broxodent Toothbrush, Squibb & Sons, Inc.
Interplak, Dental Research Corp.
Rotadent, Pro-Dentec
Sunbeam Automatic Toothbrush (Provisionally Acceptable) Northern Electric Co.
Water Pik, Teledyne Water Pik

DENTAL FLOSS

Dental Floss, John O. Butler Co.

Dental Floss, Colgate-Palmolive Co.
Dental Floss, Johnson & Johnson Professional Dental Care Co.
Floss for Kids, Johnson & Johnson Professional Dental Care Co.
Jordan Dental Floss, Jordan
Oral-B Dental Floss, Oral-B Laboratories
Oral-B Flossers, Oral-B Laboratories
Oral-B Super Floss, Oral-B Laboratories
Personal Dental Floss, Flossrite Corp.
Ranir Dental Floss (Waxed & Unwaxed), Henry Schein, Inc.

ORAL-HYGIENE AIDS

Dr. Flosser Device, Flossrite Corp.
Jordan Dental Sticks, Jordan
Oral-B Interdental Brush, Oral-B Laboratories
Orapik, Dental Concepts, Inc.
Proxabrush & Stimulator, John O. Butler Co.
Sakool Tongue Cleaner, Sakool Co.
Silverak Tongue Cleaning Device, Gautamas, Inc.
Stim-U-Dent Interdental Cleaner, Johnson & Johnson Professional Care Co.

There are many other aids to oral hygiene not listed by the ADA but recommended, nevertheless, by periodontists to meet the individual needs of patients. Some require a prescription for purchase at a pharmacy. Among those that are available over-the-counter are the following:
Perio-Aid, Marquis Dental Mfg. Co.
Butler Eez-Thru Floss Threader, John O. Butler Co.
Butler Proxabrush Traveler, John O. Butler Co.
FlossMate Floss Handle, John O. Butler Co.
Pick.A.Dent, Denticator Co. ✣

Appendix B

RECOMMENDED READING

For more information on any of the subjects discussed in this book and many more, such as teaching aids, you may write for the "ADA Catalogue" published by The American Dental Association.

American Dental Association
211 East Chicago Avenue
Chicago, Illinois 60611

It offers a large selection of short pamphlets containing up-to-date information on all aspects of dental health. Some sample titles are: *Basic Brushing; Gum Disease, Eight Silent Signs; Seal Out Decay; Complete Your Fitness Plan With Fluoride; Referral To A Dental Specialist; Your Teeth And What They Do; Keeping Your Smile In Later Years; How To Be A Wise Dental Consumer; Pregnancy And Oral Health; Your Child's Teeth; Tooth Survival Book; The Tooth Chicken; Happiness Is A Healthy Mouth; Orthodontics: Questions And Answers; Fixed Bridges And Crowns; Removable Partial Dentures; Periodontal Disease, Don't Wait Till It Hurts*; and many others.

Similar books and pamphlets are offered to dentists for distribution to their patients by many of the manufacturers of oral-hygiene aids and appliances.

Information on diet and health is available from a large selection of books and monthly newsletters. Here are some recently published books on Diet and Health selected by the editors of *Tufts University Diet and Nutrition Newsletter* that should be available in libraries and bookstores.

Take Care of Yourself, Donald M. Vickery, MD and James M. Fries, MD. (Addison-Wesley, Reading, Massachusetts. Softcover, $16.95. 800-447-2226).

The Tufts University Guide To Total Nutrition, Stanley Gershoff, PhD, with Catherine Whitney and the Editorial Advisory Board of the *Tufts University Diet and Nutrition Newsletter* (Harper & Row, New York. Hardcover, $22.50. 800-242-7737).

Food Lover's Companion, Sharon Tyler Herbst. (Barron's, Hauppauge, New York. Softcover, $10.95. 800-645-3476).

Better Homes And Gardens Low-Fat Meals. (Meredith Corporation, Des Moines, Iowa. Hardcover, $9.95. 515-284-2363, call collect).

Cooking Light Cookbook 1990, (Oxmoor House, Birmingham, Alabama. Hardcover, $19.95. 800-633-4910).

The Restaurant Companion; A Guide To Healthier Eating Out. Hope S. Warsaw, RD. (Surrey Books, Chicago, Illinois. Softcover, $11.95. 800-326-4430).

The Guiltless Gourmet Goes Ethnic, Judy Gilliard and Joy Kilpatrick, RD. (DCI Publishing, Minneapolis, Minnesota. Softcover, $11.95. 800-848-2793).

The Cook's Garden; Growing And Using The Best-Tasting Vegetable Varieties, Shepherd and Ellen Ogden. (Rodale Press, Emmaus, Pennsylvania. Hardcover, $19.95. Softcover $14.95. 800-441-7761).

Almost every large university publishes a monthly Newsletter on diet, nutrition, and health. A subscription to any one of them will be helpful in keeping up with current thinking and changes in opinion as new research is reported in the medical literature. The current surge of interest in nutrition and a healthy lifestyle has made them more profitable to the publishers and very competitive. After you subscribe to one you will hear from many others. Here are a few to choose from.

Tuft's University Diet And Nutrition Newsletter, Editor, Stanley N. Gershoff, PhD, Dean, School of Nutrition. New Subscription Information: P.O. Box 57857, Boulder, Colorado, 80322-7857; $20 per year (12 issues).

The John Hopkins Medical Letter, Health After 50, Editor/Publisher, Rodney Friedman, P.O.Box 420179, Palm Coast, Florida, 32142; $24 per year (12 issues).

Executive Health Report, Editor, Kate Kupferer, P.O. Box 8880, Chapel Hill, North Carolina, 27515; $34 per year (12 issues).

University Of California, Berkeley Wellness Letter, P.O.Box 420163, Palm Coast, Florida, 32142; $15 per year (12 issues).

It's Your Colesterol, Editor, Diane B. Stoy, RN, MA, Lipid Research Clinic, George Washington University, 2700 Prosperity Avenue, Fairfax, Virginia 22031, 800-654-7134; $19.95 per year (12 issues). ✥